REVERSING HIGH BLOOD PRESSURE
7 Natural Secrets to Safely Lower Blood Pressure

Second Edition

Dr. Joseph Jacobs, DPT, ACN

Second Edition, January 2026
Published by ASTR Institute
614 E HWY 50 #169, Clermont, FL 34711

ASTR

ASTRinstitute.com

Disclaimer

This book, authored by Dr. Joseph Jacobs and published by the ASTR Institute, is intended for informational purposes only and presents medical research findings. It is not a substitute for professional medical advice, diagnosis, or treatment. Dr. Joseph Jacobs, the ASTR Institute, and its affiliates do not endorse or assume responsibility for any specific medical treatments or procedures discussed in this book. We strongly advise readers to consult with their healthcare providers regarding the applicability of any aspects of the content to their own health and well-being.

The statements contained herein have not been evaluated by the Food and Drug Administration. The products mentioned are not designed to diagnose, cure, treat, or prevent any disease. Individual results may vary, and we cannot guarantee that you will achieve the same outcomes as those detailed in our case studies, testimonials, and treatment videos. Success varies per individual, and one person's results do not guarantee similar outcomes for another.

If you have medical concerns, consult with your healthcare provider, physician, or another qualified medical professional. Dr. Joseph Jacobs, the ASTR Institute, and their associated organizations and individuals disclaim any liability for actions, services, or products acquired through this book, our videos, website, or any of our media channels.

Table of Contents

Online Resources

How to Access Online Resources

Throughout this book, you'll find barcodes that link to additional online resources. Here's how to use them:

1. Open the camera app on your smartphone.
2. Point the camera at the barcode.
3. A notification will appear with a link. Tap the notification to open the link in your browser.

Triumph Over Trials: My Journey from Disability to Victory

After my second cancer treatment, I was suffering from chronic fatigue, migraines, muscle and joint pain. I reached out to at least seven doctors, but I could not find relief. Unfortunately, they had two responses. First, they said my blood labs looked normal. I learned from my studies in nutrition that this happened because they did not order the correct labs to figure out the root cause of my issues. The second response was that I was a hopeless case. This made me realize that if I wanted to overcome my disability, I had to look for a solution on my own. It was a difficult time in my life. Due to my pain and fatigue, it used to take me 10 minutes just to walk from the living room to the bathroom, about 20 feet away. I was very depressed and angry because, at 30 years old, I was facing numerous health issues and had a poor quality of life without any answers.

I spent countless hours and years studying nutrition, psychology, behavioral modification, anatomy, physiology, ergonomics, and other medical topics in hopes of finding an answer. At the same time, I was frustrated that the techniques I learned in medical school only provided short-term results with no lasting relief. I tried what I learned in school, such as stretching, exercises, electrical stimulation, various massage techniques, manual therapy, joint mobilization, and myofascial release, but nothing provided long-term results. So, I started to look at medical studies to guide me through this process. After reviewing over 16,000 medical research papers with assistance from medical students, I was shocked and disappointed by the results. Based on these studies, the following treatments either provided no pain reduction or only short-term pain reduction:

- NSAIDs
- Opioids
- Cortisone shots
- Exercises
- Stretching
- Massage
- Joint mobilization or manipulation
- Acupuncture
- Dry needling

- Instrument-assisted soft tissue mobilization

I have dedicated my life to researching all current traditional medical approaches to treating pain. I've found that the majority of these approaches primarily focus on relieving symptoms rather than addressing the root cause of the pain. The techniques I learned in school, still used in today's modern medical world, have their origins in ancient healing practices such as manipulation, massage, stretching, and exercise. These methods were used by the Romans, Greeks, and Egyptians to increase flexibility, strengthen muscles, and alleviate pain. Today's medicine has added treatments like cold, heat, electrical stimulation, and joint adjustment to this list. However, overwhelming evidence from published medical studies shows no promising long-term relief from any of these methods.

For instance, one systematic review conducted by the University of Ottawa, Canada, which reviewed 270 research studies, concluded that the benefits of massage, acupuncture, and spine adjustment treatments were mostly evident immediately or shortly after treatment, then faded over time. With compelling data like this, it is perplexing how we continue to treat patients with modalities that do not effectively address their long-term needs. Instead of focusing so much on the body's symptoms, we need to start questioning why these symptoms are present in the first place and why they keep returning.

This question guided me through an intense investigative research process over five years. From this research, I concluded that there are seven aspects of chronic pain that, when treated simultaneously, can lead to long-term pain relief. In my book, **Pain No More**, I outline seven key elements that must be addressed simultaneously to effectively relieve chronic pain. I also found that the BioPsychosocial model is an effective treatment approach for long-term pain reduction. So, I studied the BioPsychosocial model in depth and realized that my medical education was lacking in nutrition knowledge. I spent thousands of hours reading and studying nutrition and bought any book that I felt could help me understand the body better.

During this time, my wife had chronic jaw pain due to stress at work. I tried everything I learned from school on her, but nothing provided long-term pain relief. One day she woke up with lockjaw, unable to speak or open her mouth. She asked me to try anything. I told her that I had tried everything I knew, but nothing worked. So, I reached inside her mouth and experimented with several maneuvers. After a few minutes, she was able to open her mouth and was pain-free. I was dumbfounded and had no idea what had just happened. It took me several days to understand the physiology of the maneuvers I had performed. I then started experimenting with the same concept, applying it to the whole body to relieve both my pain and my patients' pain.

After several months of using my hands to implement the new maneuvers I had come up with, I realized I could not do that long-term. My hands were very sore, and I suffered from pain every night. I told my wife that this was not sustainable because I was in so much pain from using my hands. While patients were getting relief, I was suffering. My wife suggested that I use tools instead of my hands. So, I went to a hardware store and bought rubber, plastic, and metal to cut and design tools and devices to replace my hand maneuvers. Thankfully, this provided even faster results for my patients without me feeling soreness from working on them.

I was able to overcome my chronic fatigue and migraines by running comprehensive lab tests. These tests revealed several vitamin, mineral, and hormonal imbalances. Additionally, I overcame my chronic joint and muscle pain through the biopsychosocial (BPS) model and the tools and devices I invented. I also reinvented the biopsychosocial model to be implemented by a single healthcare provider and called it ASTR treatment.

My journey toward developing the ASTR diet was driven by personal challenges and professional insights. I experienced significant frustration with various diets that often left me feeling fatigued and unsatisfied. Through an extensive review of research studies, I also uncovered potential health risks associated with extreme dietary approaches. These experiences inspired me to create the ASTR Diet as a healthier, evidence-based alternative, which I share in my book **Eat to Heal**.

For years, I suffered from debilitating migraines, searching for lasting relief beyond temporary fixes. My journey as both a patient and a healthcare provider led me to dedicate 15 years to researching, studying, and testing effective solutions. Through this process, I developed a comprehensive approach that transformed my own health and has helped countless patients overcome chronic migraines and pain. In this book, I share these evidence-based strategies, solutions that I have refined through experience and clinical practice. My hope is that this book serves as a practical guide to empower you on your path to recovery, providing the tools and knowledge needed to reclaim a pain-free life.

Understanding High Blood Pressure (Hypertension)

High blood pressure, also known as hypertension, is a common condition in which the force of the blood against your artery walls is consistently too high. Over time, this excessive pressure can damage blood vessels and increase the risk of heart disease, stroke, kidney damage, and other serious health problems (Whelton et al., 2018).

Symptoms of High Blood Pressure:

Hypertension is often referred to as a **"silent killer"** because it typically has no obvious symptoms until significant damage has occurred. However, in some cases, individuals may experience:

- Headaches
- Dizziness
- Nosebleeds
- Shortness of breath
- Blurred vision

These symptoms are not exclusive to hypertension and usually appear only in cases of severely elevated blood pressure.

Biophysiology of Hypertension:

To understand how hypertension develops, it's essential to look at the biophysiology, or how the body's physical processes are involved. Blood pressure is determined by two main factors:

- Cardiac output (CO): the amount of blood your heart pumps per minute.
- Peripheral resistance (PR): the resistance your blood vessels offer against blood flow.

Hypertension often results from increased cardiac output, increased peripheral resistance, or both. Factors such as high sodium intake, obesity, hormonal imbalances, and chronic stress can disrupt this balance and lead to persistently elevated pressure (Carretero & Oparil, 2000).

Blood Vessels and the Endothelium:

The endothelium is a thin layer of cells lining the interior surface of blood vessels. Far from being inert, the endothelium plays a vital role in regulating vascular tone, blood flow, clotting, and immune function. It acts as a gatekeeper between the bloodstream and surrounding tissues, releasing substances such as nitric oxide (NO), which relaxes blood vessels and lowers blood pressure. When functioning properly, the endothelium supports smooth circulation and reduces inflammation. However, chronic inflammation, oxidative stress, poor diet, smoking, and high blood sugar can impair endothelial function, an early step in the development of hypertension and atherosclerosis.

Oxidative stress and chronic inflammation are two of the most damaging influences on endothelial health. Excess reactive oxygen species (ROS) degrade nitric oxide, a key molecule responsible for vasodilation and vascular protection. When nitric oxide availability is reduced, blood vessels become stiffer, more prone to clotting, and more reactive to hypertensive signals. This dysfunction marks the transition from a healthy vascular state to one of progressive cardiovascular disease. Studies have shown that oxidative stress not only damages the endothelial lining but also promotes the expression of inflammatory markers and adhesion molecules, further worsening vascular inflammation and plaque formation.

Oxidative Stress, Inflammation, and Hypertension:

Oxidative stress and chronic inflammation are central contributors to the development and progression of high blood pressure. Oxidative stress occurs when the body produces excessive reactive oxygen species (ROS) that overwhelm its natural antioxidant defenses. These unstable molecules damage proteins, lipids, and DNA and impair vascular function. In blood vessels, oxidative stress specifically reduces the bioavailability of nitric oxide, a key molecule that helps relax and dilate blood vessels. When nitric oxide levels are depleted, vascular tone increases, promoting vasoconstriction and elevating blood pressure. This biochemical imbalance sets the stage for endothelial dysfunction, which is a hallmark of hypertension and early cardiovascular disease.

Inflammation further amplifies this process. Elevated blood pressure is not merely a mechanical issue but is also driven by immune system activation. Inflammatory cytokines such as interleukin-6 (IL-6), tumor necrosis factor-alpha (TNF-α), and C-reactive protein (CRP) contribute to vascular stiffness and increase the responsiveness of blood vessels to vasoconstrictive signals. These inflammatory markers disrupt the endothelium, enhance sodium retention, and activate the sympathetic nervous system, all of which elevate blood pressure. Inflammatory signaling also promotes remodeling of the vascular wall, making arteries less elastic and more prone to injury over time.

Research supports that individuals with elevated inflammatory markers are more likely to develop hypertension and suffer adverse cardiovascular outcomes. A prospective study published in *Circulation* found that higher levels of CRP were associated with an increased risk of incident hypertension, independent of other risk factors. Furthermore, lifestyle interventions that reduce inflammation, such as adopting an anti-inflammatory diet, increasing physical activity, managing stress, and improving sleep, have been shown to lower both systemic inflammation and blood pressure. Addressing oxidative stress and inflammation at their root is essential for effective, long-term blood pressure management and cardiovascular health.

Atherosclerosis and Its Impact on Hypertension

Atherosclerosis is a chronic condition characterized by the buildup of plaque consisting of cholesterol, inflammatory cells, calcium, microplastics and fibrous tissue within arterial walls. This accumulation narrows the arteries and reduces their elasticity. As the vessels become stiffer and more constricted, the heart must work harder to circulate blood, leading to an increase in vascular resistance and elevated blood pressure (Libby et al., 2011).

In addition to raising vascular resistance, atherosclerosis damages the endothelium, the thin inner cellular lining of blood vessels, and disrupts its ability to produce nitric oxide. Nitric oxide is essential for vasodilation, a process that allows blood vessels to relax and widen. When nitric oxide production is impaired, vasoconstriction occurs more frequently, which further contributes to the development and progression of hypertension (Ghiadoni et al., 2008).

The relationship between atherosclerosis and hypertension is bidirectional. Chronic high blood pressure damages arterial walls and accelerates plaque formation. At the same time, existing atherosclerotic changes make it harder for blood to flow freely, which maintains or worsens elevated pressure. This cycle increases the risk of serious cardiovascular events, including stroke, heart attack, and kidney disease (Williams et al., 2018). Addressing both conditions simultaneously through dietary changes, physical activity, and targeted therapies is essential for reducing long-term health risks.

Types of High Blood Pressure:

There are two primary types of hypertension:

1. **Primary (Essential) Hypertension**: This type develops gradually over many years. It accounts for about 90–95% of all cases. This type of hypertension is typically caused by a combination of the seven elements presented in this book: poor nutrition, adverse medication effects, nutrient and hormonal imbalances, lack of beneficial herbal support, physical inactivity, chronic stress, and unhelpful behavioral patterns. These factors often interact and compound over time, disrupting the body's natural balance and elevating blood pressure. By identifying and addressing each of these root contributors, lasting improvements can be achieved without solely relying on medication.
2. **Secondary Hypertension**: This results from an underlying condition such as kidney disease, adrenal gland tumors, or medication side effects. It tends to appear suddenly and cause higher blood pressure levels than primary hypertension.

Blood Pressure Categories and Definitions:

The American College of Cardiology and American Heart Association define blood pressure categories as follows (Whelton et al., 2018):

- **Normal**: Systolic <120 mm Hg and Diastolic <80 mm Hg
- **Elevated**: Systolic 120–129 mm Hg and Diastolic <80 mm Hg
- **Hypertension Stage 1**: Systolic 130–139 mm Hg or Diastolic 80–89 mm Hg
- **Hypertension Stage 2**: Systolic ≥140 mm Hg or Diastolic ≥90 mm Hg

- **Hypertensive Crisis**: Systolic >180 mm Hg and/or Diastolic >120 mm Hg (requires immediate medical attention)

Systolic pressure refers to the pressure in your arteries when your heart beats, while **diastolic pressure** is the pressure in your arteries when your heart rests between beats.

Statistics

According to the Centers for Disease Control and Prevention (CDC), nearly **half of adults in the United States (47%)** have hypertension (CDC, 2023). Despite its prevalence, only 1 in 4 adults with hypertension have their condition under control. Hypertension contributes to nearly **700,000 deaths per year** in the U.S., either as a primary or contributing cause.

The condition is more common with age and tends to affect men more than women before age 55, after which women are at greater risk. It also disproportionately affects African American compared to other racial or ethnic groups.

Other Types of Hypertension:

- **White Coat Hypertension**: This occurs when a person's blood pressure readings are higher in a clinical setting than at home. It may be a stress-related response to the medical environment and does not always indicate chronic hypertension. Home monitoring or 24-hour ambulatory blood pressure testing is often recommended to confirm diagnosis.
- **Masked Hypertension**: The opposite of white coat hypertension, this is when blood pressure appears normal at the doctor's office but is elevated in daily life. It can be particularly dangerous because it often goes undetected without home monitoring.

Complications of Uncontrolled Hypertension:

- **Heart disease**: including heart failure, heart attack, arrhythmias, and myocardial infarction.
- **Stroke**: due to damage to arteries supplying the brain.

- **Kidney disease**: hypertension is a leading cause of chronic kidney disease and can accelerate kidney failure.
- **Vision loss**: damage to the tiny blood vessels in the eyes (hypertensive retinopathy).
- **Cognitive decline**: linked to an increased risk of dementia.

Monitoring Recommendations:

Adults over 18 should have their blood pressure checked at least once every 1–2 years, and more frequently if they are at risk or have a prior diagnosis.

Risk Factors for Hypertension:

Hypertension does not develop overnight. **It is typically the result of multiple risk factors, many of which are modifiable**. Understanding these factors is essential for both prevention and effective management. Some of the most common contributors include:

- **Poor Diet**: Diets high in sodium, processed foods, added sugars, and unhealthy fats contribute significantly to elevated blood pressure. Lack of nutrient-dense, whole foods further exacerbates the problem.
- **Chronic Stress**: Ongoing emotional or psychological stress can activate the body's fight or flight response, increasing heart rate and narrowing blood vessels, which raises blood pressure over time.
- **Physical Inactivity**: A sedentary lifestyle weakens the cardiovascular system and impairs circulation, both of which contribute to increased blood pressure.
- **Medication Side Effects**: Certain medications, such as decongestants, pain relievers, birth control pills, and some antidepressants, can cause or worsen hypertension.
- **Nutrient and Hormonal Imbalances**: Deficiencies in key minerals like magnesium and potassium, along with imbalances in hormones like cortisol, thyroid, and insulin, are common but often overlooked contributors to hypertension.
- **Unhealthy Behaviors**: Smoking, alcohol consumption, poor sleep habits, and inconsistent health routines can all lead to sustained elevations in blood pressure.

- **Genetics and Family History**: While you cannot change your genes, a family history of hypertension can increase your risk, especially when combined with lifestyle and environmental factors.

Addressing these root contributors through a comprehensive, natural approach, as outlined in the seven elements of this book, can significantly reduce your risk and support long-term blood pressure control.

Conclusion

Understanding what high blood pressure is and how it develops is crucial for prevention and treatment. Recognizing early signs, knowing the risk factors, and understanding the body's internal mechanisms can empower individuals to take proactive steps toward heart health.

Research Evidence

The Biopsychosocial Evidence for Reversing High Blood Pressure

High blood pressure is not a single-cause condition. It is a progressive cardiovascular disorder that develops through the interaction of biological dysfunction, psychological stress physiology, and long-standing behavioral patterns. While conventional care has focused primarily on lowering blood pressure values through medication, a substantial body of research demonstrates that blood pressure is strongly influenced by upstream, modifiable drivers. When those drivers remain unaddressed, hypertension frequently persists or progresses despite pharmacologic treatment.

Biopsychosocial Model

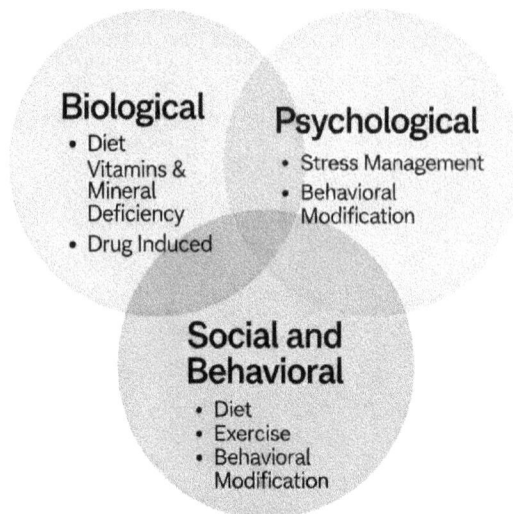

Biological
- Diet
  Vitamins &
  Mineral
  Deficiency
- Drug Induced

Psychological
- Stress Management
- Behavioral
  Modification

Social and Behavioral
- Diet
- Exercise
- Behavioral
  Modification

The Biomedical Model: Strengths and Limitations

Traditional hypertension care is largely rooted in the biomedical model, which views disease as the result of identifiable biological abnormalities that can be isolated, measured, and treated, most often through medication. Within this framework, elevated blood pressure is interpreted as a mechanical or biochemical malfunction, such as increased vascular resistance, excess fluid volume, or dysregulated renin-angiotensin signaling. The biomedical model has clear strengths. It has contributed to life-saving medications, improved acute care, and reduced cardiovascular events in high-risk populations.

However, its limitation lies in scope. By focusing primarily on biological endpoints and symptom suppression, the biomedical model often overlooks the psychological and behavioral processes that initiate, perpetuate, or worsen hypertension over time. As a result, treatment frequently centers on controlling numbers rather than addressing why those numbers became elevated in the first place. This narrow focus helps explain why many patients experience medication escalation, side effects, partial response, or resistant hypertension despite adherence to prescribed therapy.

The Biopsychosocial Model: A Systems-Based Framework

To address these limitations, the biopsychosocial model was introduced by George Engel as a more comprehensive framework for understanding chronic disease (Engel, 1977). Rather than isolating illness to a single organ system, this model recognizes that health and disease arise from the dynamic interaction of multiple systems operating simultaneously.

Within the biopsychosocial model, hypertension is shaped by:

- **Biological factors**, including inflammation, endothelial dysfunction, arterial stiffness, insulin resistance, oxidative stress, nutrient deficiencies, hormonal dysregulation, kidney sodium handling, and medication effects.
- **Psychological factors**, including chronic stress activation, anxiety, trauma exposure, autonomic nervous system imbalance, emotional regulation, and sleep disruption.
- **Social and behavioral factors**, including dietary patterns, physical activity, alcohol exposure, medication use, sleep habits, work demands, environmental stressors, and daily routines that shape long-term physiology.

Decades of clinical, behavioral, and epidemiological research support this integrated approach, demonstrating that chronic diseases are rarely the product of a single pathway (Borrell-Carrió et al., 2004).

Why Hypertension Fits the Biopsychosocial Model

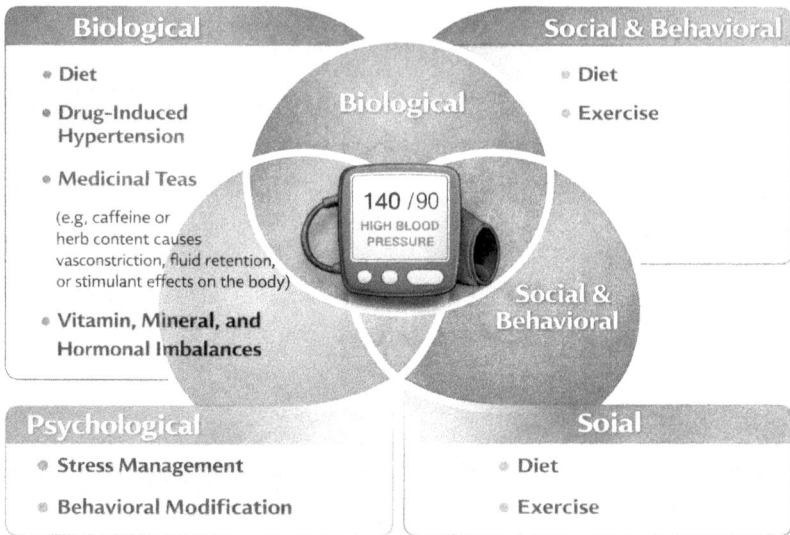

Hypertension is particularly well suited to a biopsychosocial framework because blood pressure is not a static measurement. It is a dynamic physiological output influenced by vascular function, kidney regulation, nervous system tone, hormonal signaling, metabolic health, emotional stress, and habitual behavior.

Changes in any one of these domains can raise or lower blood pressure, often independently of medication. Research consistently shows that psychological stress can elevate sympathetic nervous system activity, sleep disruption alters hormonal regulation, dietary patterns influence vascular tone and inflammation, and medications or substances can unintentionally raise blood pressure. These influences do not operate in isolation. They interact, amplify one another, and shape long-term cardiovascular regulation.

Organizing the Evidence Through a Biopsychosocial Lens

The **seven natural secrets** presented throughout this book are organized directly around this biopsychosocial structure. Each secret reflects one or more layers of the model and represents a category of evidence-supported contributors to elevated blood pressure. This chapter presents the **s**cientific evidence supporting each category within that framework. Practical strategies, protocols, and implementation are intentionally reserved for the chapters that follow. The purpose of this section is to establish that reversing high blood pressure is not a matter of opinion or lifestyle preference, but a systems-based approach grounded in decades of interdisciplinary research.

Secret One: Food-Induced Hypertension

Evidence linking nutrition to blood pressure dysregulation

Dietary intake exerts continuous influence on blood pressure through effects on vascular tone, nitric oxide availability, inflammation, insulin signaling, gut-derived metabolites, oxidative stress, and renal fluid regulation. Nutritional exposure is therefore a biological driver of hypertension, shaped by behavioral consistency over time. Large-scale reviews demonstrate that diets high in ultra-processed foods are associated with higher blood pressure and increased risk of hypertension. An umbrella review examining ultra-processed food consumption and cardiometabolic outcomes found consistent associations with hypertension, likely mediated by excess sodium, low potassium density, endothelial dysfunction, and inflammatory activation (Lane et al., 2024).

Prospective cohort evidence also links sugar-sweetened beverage consumption to incident hypertension. A systematic review and meta-analysis of cohort studies reported a significantly higher risk of developing hypertension among individuals with higher intake of sugar-sweetened beverages (Jayalath et al., 2015). These findings support mechanistic research showing that repeated glucose and fructose exposure increases uric acid production, sympathetic activity, vascular stiffness, and insulin resistance. Mineral balance further reinforces the dietary connection. A systematic review and meta-analysis found that increased potassium intake reduced blood pressure in adults with hypertension and improved cardiovascular risk markers, highlighting the role of nutrient-dense, whole-food dietary patterns in vascular regulation (Aburto et al., 2013).

Dietary patterns characterized by anti-inflammatory food selection, high polyphenol intake, fiber density, and low toxin exposure have repeatedly demonstrated blood pressure benefits. Meta-analytic evidence evaluating Mediterranean-style dietary interventions shows reductions in both systolic and diastolic blood pressure, supporting dietary frameworks that emphasize whole, unprocessed foods and metabolic restoration. These findings align closely with the foundational principles of the ASTR dietary model (Soltani et al., 2024). Within the biopsychosocial framework, food-induced hypertension reflects a biological process reinforced by behavioral repetition and environmental exposure.

Secret Two: Drug-Induced Hypertension

Evidence that medications and substances elevate blood pressure

Medication exposure is a frequently overlooked contributor to persistent or resistant hypertension. Many commonly used drugs influence blood pressure through renal sodium retention, vascular constriction, endocrine signaling, or sympathetic activation. Nonsteroidal anti-inflammatory drugs (NSAIDs) are among the most extensively studied examples. Meta-analyses have demonstrated that NSAID use is associated with measurable increases in blood pressure, particularly in individuals with pre-existing hypertension (Pope et al., 1993; Johnson et al., 1994). These effects are clinically relevant because they may also blunt the effectiveness of antihypertensive therapy.

More recent randomized evidence supports drug-specific differences. The PRECISION-ABPM trial showed that ibuprofen increased ambulatory systolic blood pressure to a greater extent than celecoxib and was associated with a higher incidence of new-onset hypertension (Ruschitzka et al., 2017).

Alcohol functions as a pharmacologically active substance with direct blood pressure effects. A large systematic review and meta-analysis demonstrated that reductions in alcohol intake produced dose-dependent decreases in blood pressure, particularly in individuals with higher baseline consumption (Roerecke et al., 2017).

Hormonal medications also contribute. A meta-analysis evaluating oral contraceptive use found a positive association between duration of use and hypertension risk, with incremental risk increases over time (Liu et al., 2017). Within the biopsychosocial model, drug-induced hypertension represents a biological pressure load that is often sustained by social norms, symptom-driven medication use, and long-term exposure patterns.

Secret Three: Medicinal Teas

Evidence for botanical effects on vascular physiology

Certain botanicals influence blood pressure through antioxidant activity, nitric oxide signaling, and endothelial function. Clinical research supports measurable physiological effects from specific medicinal teas. Hibiscus (*Hibiscus sabdariffa*) has one of the strongest evidence bases. A systematic review and meta-analysis found that hibiscus consumption was associated with significant reductions in blood pressure and improvements in cardiometabolic markers (Ellis et al., 2022). Polyphenol-rich teas, particularly green tea, have also been evaluated in randomized trials. Meta-analyses report modest but significant reductions in systolic and diastolic blood pressure associated with green tea supplementation, likely mediated by catechin-related improvements in endothelial function and oxidative stress (Xu et al., 2020; Mahdavi-Roshan et al., 2020).

Dietary nitrate exposure through plant-based beverages has also been studied. A systematic review and meta-analysis found that nitrate-rich beetroot juice lowered blood pressure in individuals with hypertension, supporting nitric oxide–dependent vasodilation as a relevant mechanism (Benjamim et al., 2022). In the biopsychosocial framework, medicinal teas represent biologically active compounds that are often integrated through behavioral rituals and daily routines.

Secret Four: Vitamin, Mineral, and Hormonal Imbalances

Evidence for micronutrient and endocrine contributions to hypertension

Blood pressure regulation depends on electrolyte balance, vascular smooth muscle function, renal handling of sodium and water, and endocrine signaling. Disruptions in these systems can produce persistent hypertension. Magnesium plays a central role in vascular tone and calcium channel regulation. A meta-analysis of randomized controlled trials found that magnesium supplementation significantly reduced blood pressure, supporting its physiological importance in endothelial and smooth muscle function (Zhang et al., 2016). Potassium is one of the most consistently validated nutrients in blood pressure research. A comprehensive systematic review and meta-analysis found that increased potassium intake reduced blood pressure in hypertensive adults without adverse effects, reinforcing its role in sodium balance and vascular relaxation (Aburto et al., 2013).

Hormonal contributors are equally significant. Primary aldosteronism, characterized by excessive aldosterone secretion and sodium retention, is increasingly recognized as a common and underdiagnosed cause of hypertension. Recent meta-analyses estimate prevalence rates near 9–10% among hypertensive populations and substantially higher in resistant hypertension (Huang et al., 2024).

Thyroid dysfunction also influences vascular resistance. Meta-analytic evidence demonstrates that subclinical hypothyroidism is associated with higher blood pressure compared with euthyroid states, reflecting altered vascular tone and metabolic regulation (Ye et al., 2014; Kim et al., 2021). Sleep-related hormonal disruption further contributes. A systematic review and meta-analysis found that short sleep duration is associated with increased risk of hypertension, highlighting the role of cortisol dysregulation and autonomic imbalance (Wang et al., 2012). This secret bridges biological and psychological layers within the biopsychosocial model, with behavioral patterns such as sleep timing reinforcing endocrine effects.

Secret Five: Exercise

Evidence that physical activity modifies blood pressure physiology

Exercise influences blood pressure through improvements in endothelial function, arterial compliance, insulin sensitivity, inflammation reduction, and autonomic nervous system balance. A major meta-analysis of randomized controlled trials found that aerobic exercise significantly reduced blood pressure in both hypertensive and normotensive adults (Whelton et al., 2002). A broader systematic review and meta-analysis confirmed that multiple forms of exercise training, including endurance, resistance, and combined modalities, are associated with blood pressure reductions (Cornelissen & Smart, 2013). Within the biopsychosocial framework, exercise reflects biological adaptation reinforced by behavioral consistency and environmental context.

Secret Six: Stress Management

Evidence that psychological stress elevates blood pressure

Chronic psychological stress produces sustained activation of the sympathetic nervous system and hypothalamic-pituitary-adrenal axis, increasing vascular resistance, cortisol levels, and blood pressure variability. Meta-analyses of randomized controlled trials indicate that mindfulness-based stress reduction and related interventions are associated with reductions in blood pressure among individuals with elevated blood pressure or hypertension (Lee et al., 2020). More recent systematic reviews continue to support these associations while emphasizing the physiological impact of stress modulation on cardiovascular outcomes (Mir et al., 2024). This body of evidence confirms that psychological regulation is inseparable from biological blood pressure control.

Secret Seven: Behavioral Modification

Evidence that sustained behavior shapes long-term blood pressure outcomes

Hypertension is strongly influenced by daily behavior patterns that determine cumulative physiological load. Research consistently shows stronger outcomes when multiple lifestyle behaviors are addressed together. The PREMIER trial demonstrated that comprehensive lifestyle modification produced significant blood pressure improvements compared with minimal intervention, supporting an integrated behavioral approach (Appel et al., 2003).

Self-monitoring also alters outcomes. A meta-analysis of randomized trials found that home blood pressure monitoring improved blood pressure control compared with usual care, highlighting the role of feedback and behavioral awareness (Cappuccio et al., 2004). Sleep behavior is another critical factor. Meta-analytic evidence links short sleep duration with increased hypertension risk, reinforcing sleep as a behavioral driver of autonomic and endocrine regulation (Wang et al., 2012). Within the biopsychosocial model, behavioral modification represents the social and environmental context through which biological and psychological factors are either reinforced or corrected.

Conclusion: A Scientific Model, Not Opinion

The research presented in this chapter demonstrates that high blood pressure is driven by interconnected biological, psychological, and behavioral mechanisms. Food exposure, medication effects, nutrient and hormonal balance, physical activity, stress physiology, and daily behavior patterns all contribute measurably to blood pressure regulation.The biopsychosocial model provides the unifying framework that explains why isolated interventions often fail and why a systems-based approach is required for lasting change. The chapters that follow translate this evidence into focused, practical strategies for each of the seven natural secrets, building directly on the research foundation established here.

The Roadmap to Healing

If you're holding this book, it's likely because you're ready for a real and lasting solution, not just another temporary fix. You're tired of managing symptoms with medications that only mask the problem. You're ready to address the root causes of hypertension and reclaim control over your health. This chapter lays the foundation for what's ahead and introduces the roadmap that will guide you through your healing journey.

High blood pressure (hypertension) is not a random occurrence. In most cases, it develops gradually, fueled by a combination of diet, environmental exposures, lifestyle habits, stress, and imbalances in the body. Conventional medicine often focuses on managing blood pressure through medication alone, but this approach rarely addresses the underlying issues. To experience true and lasting reversal of hypertension, we must dig deeper and correct the dysfunction at its core.

To truly get to the root of hypertension, **you must implement all seven elements presented in this book.** Each one addresses a different cause or contributor to high blood pressure. Ignoring even one may prevent full healing and leave you stuck managing symptoms rather than resolving them. These elements are not optional or interchangeable. They are interconnected, and together, they form the foundation for long-term health transformation. Below is a summary of each element with practical steps to begin applying them. This book presents seven natural elements, that must be addressed together to reverse high blood pressure effectively and sustainably:

1. Food-Induced Hypertension

Your food choices are among the most powerful tools for reversing high blood pressure or one of its greatest drivers. Diets high in refined carbohydrates, added sugars, processed meats, and inflammatory oils promote vascular inflammation, insulin resistance, and water retention, all of which elevate blood pressure. Many patients unknowingly consume foods they are sensitive or allergic to, triggering chronic immune responses that worsen hypertension. By eliminating inflammatory foods and adopting a nutrient-dense, anti-inflammatory eating pattern, such as the ASTR Diet detailed in *Eat to Heal*, you can reduce inflammation, support arterial health, and begin to restore normal blood pressure from the inside out.

2. Drug-Induced Hypertension

Many common prescription and over-the-counter medications can silently elevate blood pressure. Decongestants, nonsteroidal anti-inflammatory drugs (NSAIDs), birth control pills, certain antidepressants, and even herbal supplements can disrupt cardiovascular function or hormone balance. Unfortunately, most patients are unaware of these side effects. A thorough review of your medication list with a healthcare provider is essential. Identifying and, when appropriate, replacing or eliminating medications that contribute to hypertension is a critical step in treating the root cause rather than simply masking the symptoms.

3. Vitamin, Mineral, and Hormonal Imbalances

Micronutrient deficiencies are frequently overlooked in traditional care, yet they play a central role in blood pressure regulation. Magnesium, potassium, vitamin D, B-complex vitamins, and others all contribute to vascular tone, electrolyte balance, and stress response. From my clinical experience, most patients with hypertension have four to eight deficiencies contributing to their condition. Hormonal imbalances, such as elevated cortisol or disrupted thyroid function, can also elevate blood pressure.

4. Medicinal Teas

Certain herbal teas can be a gentle and effective way to support blood pressure reduction. Teas like hibiscus, green tea, oolong, rooibos, chamomile, and lemon balm contain plant compounds that relax blood vessels, reduce oxidative stress, and lower inflammation. Clinical studies have shown that daily consumption of hibiscus tea, in particular, can produce measurable reductions in systolic and diastolic pressure. These teas are not a replacement for other interventions, but they can serve as powerful allies in your daily routine, especially when used alongside a healthy diet and lifestyle.

5. Exercise

Physical activity is one of the most effective and immediate tools for lowering blood pressure. Regular movement improves circulation, enhances nitric oxide production, reduces arterial stiffness, and supports weight loss. Exercise does not have to be extreme or exhausting. Walking, resistance training, yoga, and even simple home-based routines can yield significant benefits when done consistently. The key is to create a plan that is enjoyable and sustainable. As you move your body, you help regulate your heart rate, manage stress hormones, and strengthen the cardiovascular system from the ground up.

6. Stress Management

Chronic stress activates the body's fight-or-flight response, increasing levels of cortisol and adrenaline, which constrict blood vessels and raise blood pressure. Over time, unrelieved stress contributes to inflammation, sleep disruption, hormonal imbalance, and unhealthy coping behaviors. Managing stress is not just a mental health strategy. It is a critical pillar of cardiovascular health. Techniques such as mindfulness, deep breathing, journaling, prayer, gratitude, and guided relaxation can all lower sympathetic nervous system activity and promote healing. When emotional roots of stress are also addressed, the body can finally shift from survival mode into a state of restoration.

7. Behavioral Modification

Lasting blood pressure reversal requires lasting behavior change. Without modifying habits, even the best diet or supplement plan will fall short. Behavioral modification involves identifying unhealthy patterns, such as poor sleep routines, excessive screen time, sedentary behavior, or emotional eating, and replacing them with intentional, health-supportive actions. Small, consistent changes add up to transformational results over time. By retraining your brain and reshaping your routines, you create the lifestyle foundation needed for long-term blood pressure control.

Each of these elements represents a major pillar of your healing. While it might be tempting to focus on just one or two areas that feel more convenient or familiar, doing so will only provide partial results. You cannot pick and choose. Hypertension is a multifactorial condition, and if you want lasting results, you must address all seven elements as part of a complete lifestyle transformation.

This is not a quick fix. Reversing hypertension naturally requires intention, commitment, and a willingness to change your habits and mindset. But the payoff is worth it. You will experience better energy, sharper focus, reduced reliance on medications, and lower risk of stroke, heart disease, and kidney failure. Most importantly, you gain the ability to take back control over your own health. In the chapters that follow, you'll learn how to identify and eliminate the root causes of high blood pressure using evidence-based tools and strategies. Each section offers practical guidance, clinical insights, and action steps you can begin implementing immediately. Let this roadmap be your guide. Healing is possible, but only if you're ready to follow the path with consistency and courage.

Conclusion: Commit to the Full Path

Reversing high blood pressure is not about shortcuts. It is about addressing the real, underlying causes with intention, consistency, and a comprehensive approach. This book outlines seven elements: food, medications, nutrient and hormonal balance, teas, exercise, stress management, and behavioral change. These components work together as an integrated system. Each one plays a vital role in restoring balance, healing the body, and lowering blood pressure naturally.

It is essential to understand that you cannot treat hypertension effectively by focusing on just one or two of these areas. True healing comes from implementing all seven elements as a cohesive lifestyle. While that may sound challenging at first, this journey is not about perfection. It is about progress. Small, steady steps in each area will build momentum and create sustainable change over time.

You are not simply managing a condition. You are transforming your health at the root. Commit fully to the process. Give your body the tools it needs to heal. And remember, you are not alone. Use the guidance in each chapter as a step forward on your roadmap to a healthier, stronger, and more vibrant life, free from the burden of high blood pressure.

Food-Induced Hypertension

Hypertension, or high blood pressure, is influenced by a wide range of factors, with diet being one of the most significant. While some foods can help regulate blood pressure, others can raise it substantially, especially when consumed frequently. This chapter explores common food-based contributors to high blood pressure, supported by clinical research and real-world case observations.

Processed Foods and Sodium

Processed foods are one of the most significant dietary contributors to high blood pressure. They are often high in sodium, low in essential nutrients, and filled with additives that disrupt the body's natural balance. Research consistently shows a strong correlation between processed food consumption and elevated blood pressure.

One of the primary concerns with processed foods is their high sodium content. Sodium causes the body to retain fluid, increasing blood volume and placing more pressure on artery walls. A large meta-analysis of randomized controlled trials found that reducing salt intake leads to meaningful decreases in both systolic and diastolic blood pressure, especially in individuals with hypertension (He et al., 2013).

In addition to sodium, ultra-processed foods contain preservatives, emulsifiers, and artificial ingredients that negatively affect cardiovascular health. A population-based study found that each 10% increase in calorie intake from ultra-processed foods was associated with a 20% greater risk of developing hypertension (Rauber et al., 2018). This is concerning, given the growing reliance on processed convenience foods in modern diets.

These foods also lack essential minerals like potassium and magnesium, which help regulate blood pressure and relax blood vessel walls. Diets low in these minerals have been independently linked to a higher risk of hypertension (Houston, 2011). Furthermore, food additives such as phosphates and nitrates can contribute to endothelial dysfunction, which impairs blood vessel flexibility and further elevates blood pressure (Fardet & Rock, 2021).

Avoiding processed foods and replacing them with fresh, whole, and nutrient-dense options is a foundational step in reversing high blood pressure. Whole foods not only reduce sodium intake but also supply the body with the vitamins, minerals, and antioxidants needed for cardiovascular health.

Refined Carbohydrates and Sugary Foods

Refined carbohydrates and sugary foods are key dietary culprits in the development and progression of high blood pressure. These foods spike blood sugar levels, increase insulin resistance, trigger inflammation, and disrupt the delicate hormonal and metabolic systems that regulate vascular function. Over time, these effects can lead to persistent elevation in blood pressure and greater cardiovascular risk.

Unlike whole carbohydrates that contain fiber and nutrients, refined carbs such as white bread, pastries, and sweetened cereals lack nutritional value and are rapidly digested. This rapid digestion causes spikes in blood glucose and insulin. Chronically high insulin levels, in turn, promote sodium retention by the kidneys, increase sympathetic nervous system activity, and stimulate vascular smooth muscle growth, all of which raise blood pressure. A large prospective study published in the *American Journal of Clinical Nutrition* found that diets with a high glycemic load were significantly associated with increased risk of hypertension (Liu et al., 2000).

Sugary beverages and processed sweets also contribute to endothelial dysfunction and oxidative stress, two key drivers of hypertension. A 15-year cohort study in the United States showed that participants who consumed more than one sugar-sweetened beverage per day had a higher risk of developing high blood pressure compared to those who consumed less than one per month (Brown et al., 2011). Excessive fructose intake, particularly from high-fructose corn syrup, has also been shown to increase uric acid levels, impair nitric oxide production, and promote inflammation. These effects impair normal vascular relaxation and contribute to elevated blood pressure (Johnson et al., 2007).

Refined carbohydrates and added sugars offer no health benefit and can silently fuel the mechanisms behind hypertension. Reducing or eliminating these foods while emphasizing whole, fiber-rich carbohydrates can improve insulin sensitivity, reduce inflammation, and support healthy blood pressure regulation.

Alcohol

Contrary to the long-held belief that moderate alcohol consumption may be safe or even beneficial, emerging research has firmly established that **no level of alcohol consumption is safe**. A comprehensive study published in *The Lancet* (GBD 2016 Alcohol Collaborators, 2018) reviewed data from 195 countries and concluded that **the safest level of alcohol consumption is zero**, as even small amounts increase the risk of cancer and other serious health issues. Alcohol is classified as a Group 1 carcinogen by the World Health Organization, meaning it is a known cause of cancer in humans. Regular intake, even at moderate levels, has been linked to cancers of the breast, esophagus, liver, colon, and mouth.

In addition to its carcinogenic effects, alcohol contributes significantly to the development of hypertension. Alcohol raises blood pressure through mechanisms such as increased sympathetic nervous system activity, oxidative stress, and arterial stiffness. A meta-analysis published in the *Journal of the American Heart Association* (Roerecke et al., 2017) found a clear dose-response relationship between alcohol consumption and elevated blood pressure. This reinforces the conclusion that even low levels of drinking can contribute to hypertension.

Alcohol is also a major driver of non-alcoholic fatty liver disease (NAFLD) and alcoholic fatty liver. Both conditions can progress to cirrhosis and liver failure. The liver must process alcohol as a toxin, and regular consumption leads to fat accumulation, inflammation, and scarring. Over time, this can compromise liver function and increase the risk of liver cancer. These findings highlight the importance of eliminating alcohol intake for those seeking to prevent or manage chronic conditions such as high blood pressure, liver disease, and cancer.

Alcohol consumption significantly contributes to elevated blood pressure and cardiovascular risk. Regular alcohol intake can cause long-term elevations in blood pressure by stimulating sympathetic nervous system activity, impairing vascular function, and causing hormonal imbalances. A study by Fuchs et al. (2001) found a strong correlation between alcohol consumption and the onset of hypertension, especially when intake exceeds one to two drinks daily.

A meta-analysis by Roerecke et al. (2017) demonstrated that reducing alcohol intake can significantly lower blood pressure, emphasizing the importance of abstinence. Both alcohol consumption and smoking are major contributors to elevated blood pressure and increased cardiovascular risk. Regular alcohol use may raise blood pressure over time by stimulating the sympathetic nervous system, impairing vascular function, and disrupting hormonal balance.

Trans Fat

Trans fats are one of the most harmful substances in the modern diet. Found in margarine, shortening, baked goods, fried foods, and many processed snacks, trans fats are created through the industrial hydrogenation of vegetable oils. These synthetic fats have been consistently linked to inflammation, arterial stiffness, and endothelial dysfunction, all of which contribute to the development of high blood pressure.

Trans fats increase low-density lipoprotein (LDL) cholesterol, reduce high-density lipoprotein (HDL) cholesterol, and promote systemic inflammation. These changes damage blood vessels and impair their ability to relax and expand properly, leading to increased vascular resistance and elevated blood pressure. A cross-sectional analysis of data from the National Health and Nutrition Examination Survey (NHANES) found that higher dietary intake of trans fats was associated with a greater prevalence of hypertension among U.S. adults (Mozaffarian et al., 2004).

Additionally, trans fats have been shown to increase the production of inflammatory markers such as C-reactive protein (CRP), which is associated with both cardiovascular disease and hypertension. In a study published in the *New England Journal of Medicine*, researchers found that women with the highest intake of trans fats had significantly higher levels of CRP and were at increased risk for cardiovascular events (Lopez-Garcia et al., 2005).

Because of their damaging effects, many countries have banned or restricted the use of industrial trans fats in food production. However, trace amounts still exist in some processed products, and misleading labeling may describe products as "0 grams trans fat" if the amount is under 0.5 grams per serving. Even small amounts consumed regularly can contribute to cumulative vascular damage over time. Eliminating trans fats from the diet is an essential step in reducing inflammation, improving arterial function, and supporting long-term blood pressure control.

Caffeine

Caffeine is one of the most widely consumed stimulants in the world. Found in coffee, tea, energy drinks, sodas, and chocolate, caffeine can temporarily raise blood pressure by stimulating the nervous system and narrowing blood vessels. While moderate intake may be safe for many people, individuals with high blood pressure or caffeine sensitivity may experience more pronounced cardiovascular effects.

Caffeine increases the release of adrenaline, which activates the body's fight-or-flight response. This can lead to a short-term rise in heart rate and blood pressure. A meta-analysis of randomized controlled trials found that caffeine consumption can increase systolic blood pressure by an average of 8 mmHg and diastolic pressure by 6 mmHg in the hours following intake (Noordzij et al., 2005). Although these effects are usually temporary, regular high consumption may contribute to sustained hypertension in sensitive individuals.

Genetic variability plays a significant role in how caffeine affects blood pressure. Some people metabolize caffeine more slowly due to variations in the CYP1A2 gene. These slow metabolizers may experience longer-lasting spikes in blood pressure and greater cardiovascular strain compared to fast metabolizers. A study published in *The Journal of the American Medical Association* found that individuals with the slow-metabolizing variant who drank two or more cups of coffee per day had a higher risk of heart attack (Cornelis et al., 2006).

Additives and Preservatives

Additives and preservatives are commonly used in processed and packaged foods to extend shelf life, enhance flavor, and improve texture. While these substances may improve the appearance and convenience of food, they can have negative consequences for cardiovascular health, particularly blood pressure regulation. Many additives interfere with normal vascular function, promote inflammation, and disrupt hormonal balance, which contributes to the development of hypertension.

Phosphates, which are frequently added to deli meats, processed cheeses, baked goods, and sodas, have been shown to impair kidney function and alter calcium metabolism. Both of these effects influence blood pressure. Excessive phosphate intake has also been linked to vascular calcification and arterial stiffness. A review published in *Advances in Nutrition* emphasized the association between high dietary phosphate and increased cardiovascular risk, including hypertension (Calvo & Uribarri, 2013).

Monosodium glutamate (MSG), a flavor enhancer found in many savory processed foods, may also contribute to elevated blood pressure. A population study conducted in China found a positive correlation between MSG consumption and systolic and diastolic blood pressure, independent of total sodium intake (He et al., 2011). While the effects may vary between individuals, especially those with underlying sensitivities, the findings support limiting MSG in those at risk for hypertension.

Nitrites and nitrates, commonly used as preservatives in processed meats such as bacon, sausage, and ham, have also been associated with endothelial dysfunction. Although naturally occurring nitrates in vegetables may have beneficial effects, synthetic nitrates used in preserved meats are often combined with other substances that create harmful nitrosamines during digestion. These compounds can damage the inner lining of blood vessels, reduce nitric oxide availability, and impair vasodilation.

Artificial sweeteners and emulsifiers found in diet foods, sugar-free snacks, and low-fat dressings have been shown in some studies to alter gut microbiota, which plays a role in metabolic and vascular health. Disruptions in gut bacteria can increase inflammation and insulin resistance, both of which contribute to elevated blood pressure (Fardet & Rock, 2021). Avoiding processed foods and focusing on whole, natural ingredients reduces exposure to these harmful additives and supports the body's natural ability to regulate blood pressure. This is a critical part of any long-term hypertension reversal strategy.

Pasteurized Dairy and Casein Sensitivity

While dairy products are often promoted as sources of calcium and protein, growing evidence suggests that pasteurized dairy can contribute to inflammation, immune reactions, and elevated blood pressure in individuals who are sensitive to its components. One of the most common culprits is casein, a protein found in milk that may trigger an inflammatory response in certain individuals. Sensitivity to casein can lead to systemic inflammation, which is a recognized contributor to hypertension.

Pasteurization, the process used to heat milk and kill harmful bacteria, also alters the structure of proteins and enzymes in dairy. These changes may reduce digestibility and increase the likelihood of immune responses, particularly in those with compromised gut integrity. A study published in the *Journal of Nutrition and Metabolism* suggested that dairy intolerance can elevate markers of inflammation and contribute to increased vascular resistance, which may raise blood pressure in susceptible individuals (Wasilewska et al., 2017).

Casein sensitivity, especially to the A1 beta-casein variant found in most conventional cow's milk, has also been linked to adverse cardiovascular effects. A clinical trial comparing A1 and A2 casein showed that participants consuming A1 casein had higher levels of inflammation and lower levels of glutathione, a key antioxidant that protects blood vessels from oxidative damage (Jianqin et al., 2016). These effects can impair endothelial function, making it more difficult for blood vessels to relax and regulate pressure effectively.

Furthermore, dairy products may contain residual hormones and antibiotics, which can interfere with the body's natural hormonal balance and contribute to fluid retention, both of which are known to influence blood pressure. While some people tolerate raw or fermented dairy better, others benefit from eliminating dairy entirely to reduce inflammation and support cardiovascular health. Identifying and removing food sensitivities such as casein can be a crucial step in addressing the root causes of hypertension.

Dehydration and Electrolyte Imbalance

Proper hydration and electrolyte balance are critical for maintaining healthy blood pressure. When the body is dehydrated, the blood becomes more concentrated, reducing overall blood volume and prompting the body to release hormones such as vasopressin and aldosterone. These hormones signal the kidneys to retain sodium and water, which causes blood vessels to constrict and blood pressure to rise.

Even mild dehydration can activate the sympathetic nervous system and increase vascular resistance. A study published in the journal *Hypertension* found that dehydration can cause measurable increases in blood pressure, especially when combined with other stressors such as heat or physical activity (Kenney et al., 2014). Dehydration also reduces the body's ability to regulate temperature and detoxify, further straining cardiovascular function.

Electrolytes such as sodium, potassium, magnesium, and calcium play essential roles in fluid regulation, nerve transmission, and muscle function. An imbalance in these minerals, particularly low potassium or magnesium levels, can impair the ability of blood vessels to relax and maintain proper tone. Inadequate potassium intake has been consistently linked to increased blood pressure and higher cardiovascular risk. Data from the National Health and Nutrition Examination Survey (NHANES) show that higher potassium intake is associated with lower blood pressure levels in both hypertensive and normotensive individuals (Cogswell et al., 2012).

Magnesium deficiency is another overlooked contributor. Magnesium helps regulate vascular tone, supports electrolyte transport, and influences over 300 enzymatic reactions. A meta-analysis of randomized trials found that magnesium supplementation significantly reduces both systolic and diastolic blood pressure, particularly in individuals with preexisting hypertension (Zhang et al., 2016). Maintaining hydration with pure water and consuming a diet rich in potassium- and magnesium-containing whole foods, including leafy greens, avocados, bananas, and nuts, can help correct imbalances and support optimal blood pressure control. Proper hydration and electrolyte balance are foundational for vascular health and should not be overlooked in any natural strategy for reversing hypertension.

Smoking

Smoking introduces nicotine and other harmful chemicals that cause immediate and sustained increases in blood pressure by constricting blood vessels, accelerating arterial stiffness, and promoting inflammation. According to Virdis et al. (2010), smokers have significantly higher blood pressure levels and an increased risk of developing chronic hypertension compared to non-smokers. Quitting smoking not only reduces blood pressure but also dramatically decreases the risk of heart disease and stroke, emphasizing the importance of smoking cessation for long-term cardiovascular health.

Many individuals with high blood pressure unknowingly consume multiple dietary triggers on a regular basis. Identifying and reducing these foods is essential for sustainable blood pressure management. A food journal and elimination strategy, removing suspect foods and observing blood pressure trends, can be a powerful tool in discovering personal dietary triggers.

Food Allergies and High Blood Pressure

An often-overlooked contributor to elevated blood pressure is food allergy or sensitivity. Many individuals suffer from mild or delayed food allergies without realizing it, and these immune reactions can lead to systemic inflammation, vascular stress, and fluctuations in blood pressure. Unlike classic allergic responses such as hives or anaphylaxis, food sensitivities may trigger subtler effects such as increased heart rate, vascular constriction, and activation of stress hormones like cortisol. These factors can contribute to elevated blood pressure over time.

A study by El-Serag et al. (2005) highlighted the inflammatory nature of food sensitivities and their potential role in gastrointestinal and cardiovascular disorders. Another study by Jackson et al. (2018) found that chronic low-grade inflammation, which can be triggered by food sensitivities, contributes to endothelial dysfunction, a key mechanism in the development of hypertension.

This connection between food-driven immune responses and blood pressure regulation underscores the need for greater awareness of hidden food triggers. Unfortunately, most people are unaware that they have food allergies, and even fewer realize that these reactions could be affecting their cardiovascular health.

As a result, they may continue consuming foods that trigger inflammation and elevate blood pressure, despite trying other interventions like exercise or medication. Keeping a detailed food and symptom journal, including notes on gluten, dairy, soy, eggs, or corn, can help uncover hidden influences and guide effective dietary changes.

From my clinical experience, I've observed a clear connection between food sensitivities and blood pressure spikes, both in my patients and in my own health. Personally, when I consume foods I'm allergic or sensitive to, such as caffeine, vanilla, or pineapple, I consistently experience a headache followed by a noticeable increase in my systolic blood pressure. It often rises by 20 points or more. These reactions are not isolated incidents but repeatable patterns that highlight the inflammatory and vascular stress triggered by food sensitivities.

This response likely occurs because the immune system becomes activated, which increases inflammation and raises stress hormones like cortisol and adrenaline. These physiological changes constrict blood vessels and impair endothelial function, making it more difficult for the body to regulate blood pressure effectively. Identifying and eliminating personal food triggers can be a powerful and natural way to lower blood pressure and improve overall vascular health. For this reason, I strongly encourage patients to track their symptoms and blood pressure in relation to their diet and to consider an elimination protocol like the ASTR Diet to support long-term healing.

How to Identify Your Personal High Blood Pressure Triggers:

Since high blood pressure is influenced by many individualized factors, it is essential to systematically test and identify which foods may be contributing to your elevated blood pressure. Many people have more than three food-related blood pressure triggers, making it important to approach the process with patience and a structured plan. Below are practical steps to help pinpoint and eliminate foods that may be worsening your blood pressure.

1. Keep a Detailed Food and Blood Pressure Journal:

Tracking what you eat and how your blood pressure responds is one of the most effective ways to identify potential dietary triggers. Use a notebook or a mobile app to record:
- Everything you eat and drink, including portion sizes and ingredients
- The time of day each meal or snack is consumed
- Blood pressure readings taken before and after meals, when possible
- Other factors such as stress levels, hydration, sleep quality, and physical activity

Over time, patterns may emerge that help link certain foods or habits to spikes in blood pressure.

2. ASTR Diet: Try an Elimination Diet

The ASTR Diet helps identify and eliminate food-based blood pressure triggers while promoting long-term healing through an anti-inflammatory, toxin-free, and restorative approach. An elimination diet is an effective method for uncovering food-related hypertension contributors and improving cardiovascular health. To follow the ASTR elimination diet effectively:

1. Remove all potential blood pressure triggers at once for a set period (typically 3–4 days). This includes processed meats, refined carbohydrates, alcohol, caffeine, artificial sweeteners, MSG, high-sodium foods, pasteurized dairy, and trans fats.
2. Focus on whole, unprocessed foods that nourish the body and support vascular health. Prioritize fresh vegetables, clean proteins, healthy fats, and nutrient-dense options.
3. Reintroduce foods systematically after the elimination phase. If blood pressure improves after 3–4 days, begin adding back one eliminated food at a time, waiting at least 1–2 days before introducing another.
4. Monitor your blood pressure readings closely. If blood pressure rises significantly after reintroducing a food, that item may be a trigger and should be avoided or limited long-term.

Following the ASTR Diet's elimination strategy helps individuals uncover their unique dietary triggers for hypertension and take proactive steps to heal naturally while supporting vascular and metabolic health. Because the ASTR Diet involves a detailed approach, it's difficult to fully explain its implementation in just a few pages. For a complete guide to using the ASTR Diet to support blood pressure control and overall health, refer to my book **Eat to Heal**.

3. Test Each Food Individually

Instead of removing multiple foods at once, some people prefer to test foods one by one to observe their effect on blood pressure. To do this:
Choose a food from the list of common high blood pressure triggers and eat a small amount. Measure your blood pressure 1–2 hours after eating, and again at your usual times. If no change occurs, try gradually increasing the portion size over a few days. If blood pressure rises or symptoms like headaches or fatigue appear, stop that food and wait a few days before testing another

4. Be Cautious When Testing Dairy

Pasteurized dairy can be difficult to assess because reactions vary by individual and product type. If you suspect dairy may be a blood pressure trigger:

• Start with small amounts of dairy, such as a tablespoon of yogurt or a few bites of cheese
• Note whether different forms (milk, cheese, yogurt) affect your blood pressure
• Some individuals react only to pasteurized dairy and tolerate raw dairy better, suggesting a sensitivity to heat-induced protein changes or processing methods
• Some people tolerate goat's or sheep's milk better than cow's milk

5. Consider Other Lifestyle Factors

Food triggers often interact with stress, hydration, poor sleep, or hormonal changes, making it hard to isolate a single cause. When testing foods, try to maintain consistency in sleep, stress levels, and hydration to get clearer results.

Conclusion

Most people with diet-related high blood pressure have more than three triggers, so identifying and eliminating just one may not be enough to see results. A systematic testing approach can help you build a personalized, heart-healthy diet. Though the process takes time, it can lead to significant improvements in blood pressure control, energy levels, and long-term cardiovascular wellness. If you're struggling to identify your triggers, working with a clinical nutritionist familiar with the ASTR Diet can provide valuable support.

Through years of research and clinical practice, I developed the ASTR Diet, a comprehensive nutritional approach designed to reduce inflammation, balance hormones, and support gut and brain health. The ASTR Diet focuses on anti-inflammatory, sustainable, toxin-free, and restorative foods to help the body heal naturally. It emphasizes whole, nutrient-dense foods such as organic vegetables, proteins, healthy fats, and fiber-rich carbohydrates while eliminating inflammatory foods like processed sugars, refined grains, artificial additives, and inflammatory oils.

Because the ASTR Diet is a complete lifestyle approach, it is difficult to cover all aspects in this chapter. For a detailed breakdown of the ASTR Diet and how it supports blood pressure, check out my book *Eat to Heal*, where I provide a step-by-step guide to using food as medicine to reduce inflammation, balance brain chemistry, and restore overall well-being.

EAT TO HEAL

The ASTR Diet: Unlock the Healing Power
of Food to End Sickness and Thrive

- Achieve Lasting Weight Loss
- Reverse Chronic Diseases Naturally
- Heal Inflammation and Pain
- Boost Energy and Vitality
- 3 Steps to Transform Your Health

Dr. Joseph Jacobs, DPT, ACN

Drug-Induced Hypertension

High blood pressure, or hypertension, can result not only from lifestyle factors and genetics but also as a side effect of certain medications. Understanding how drugs can induce or exacerbate hypertension is essential, particularly for individuals already managing high blood pressure. This chapter reviews medications commonly associated with elevated blood pressure and includes supporting scientific studies.

1. Nonsteroidal Anti-Inflammatory Drugs (NSAIDs)

Nonsteroidal anti-inflammatory drugs, commonly known as NSAIDs, are widely used for pain relief, inflammation, and fever reduction. Medications in this category include ibuprofen, naproxen, and diclofenac. Although they are readily available over the counter and often perceived as safe, frequent use of NSAIDs can raise blood pressure and increase the risk of cardiovascular complications, especially in individuals with preexisting hypertension.

NSAIDs interfere with the body's ability to regulate kidney function by inhibiting cyclooxygenase (COX) enzymes. This inhibition reduces the production of prostaglandins, compounds that help dilate blood vessels and maintain blood flow to the kidneys. When prostaglandin levels drop, blood vessels constrict and the kidneys retain sodium and water. This leads to an increase in blood volume and vascular resistance, which can elevate blood pressure.

A study published in the *Archives of Internal Medicine* found that regular NSAID use was associated with a significant increase in the risk of developing hypertension, particularly among women who took these medications frequently (Forman et al., 2005). Another large-scale analysis concluded that NSAID use can raise systolic blood pressure by up to 5 mmHg in patients with hypertension, potentially undermining the effectiveness of antihypertensive medications (Johnson et al., 1994).

In addition to raising blood pressure, NSAIDs may impair the function of blood pressure medications, such as ACE inhibitors, diuretics, and beta-blockers. This drug interaction can make it more difficult to achieve and maintain optimal blood pressure control. Long-term use may also increase the risk of heart attack, stroke, and kidney damage.

For individuals dealing with chronic pain or inflammation, it is important to explore safer alternatives that do not compromise cardiovascular health. These may include anti-inflammatory diets, targeted supplements, and natural pain relief strategies. Avoiding unnecessary NSAID use is a critical part of protecting long-term vascular health and reversing hypertension.

2. Decongestants

Decongestants are commonly used to relieve nasal congestion caused by colds, allergies, and sinus infections. While effective at reducing swelling in the nasal passages, these medications can have unintended consequences for individuals with high blood pressure. Many over-the-counter decongestants contain active ingredients such as pseudoephedrine or phenylephrine, which are known to constrict blood vessels throughout the body, not just in the sinuses.

These compounds work by stimulating alpha-adrenergic receptors, which leads to vasoconstriction, or the narrowing of blood vessels. Although this effect helps open nasal passages, it also raises vascular resistance and can increase both systolic and diastolic blood pressure. This makes decongestants particularly risky for individuals with existing hypertension, heart disease, or other cardiovascular risk factors.

A study published in *The American Journal of Medicine* found that pseudoephedrine significantly increased blood pressure and heart rate in individuals with controlled hypertension (Gustafson et al., 1989). Even in healthy adults, regular or high-dose use of decongestants can elevate blood pressure, especially when combined with caffeine or other stimulants.

Decongestants may also reduce the effectiveness of certain blood pressure medications and increase the likelihood of heart palpitations, anxiety, and sleep disturbances. These side effects can further strain the cardiovascular system and disrupt blood pressure regulation.

Safer alternatives for relieving congestion include steam inhalation, saline nasal sprays, anti-inflammatory foods, and herbal remedies such as eucalyptus or peppermint oil. Individuals with hypertension should always consult their healthcare provider before using decongestants, especially if symptoms persist or require long-term management.

3. Corticosteroids

Corticosteroids are anti-inflammatory medications commonly prescribed for conditions such as asthma, autoimmune diseases, allergies, skin disorders, and joint pain. While they can provide rapid symptom relief, long-term or frequent use of corticosteroids can contribute to elevated blood pressure and increase the risk of cardiovascular complications.

Corticosteroids affect blood pressure through several mechanisms. They promote sodium and water retention by the kidneys, which increases blood volume and raises blood pressure. At the same time, they enhance the sensitivity of blood vessels to circulating hormones like norepinephrine and angiotensin II, both of which cause vasoconstriction. This combination of increased fluid volume and vascular resistance creates a significant strain on the cardiovascular system.

A study published in *The Lancet* found that patients on chronic corticosteroid therapy had a significantly higher risk of developing hypertension compared to those not using these medications (Walker et al., 1994). Even low-dose, long-term corticosteroid use has been shown to increase blood pressure and impair endothelial function, which reduces the ability of blood vessels to dilate and regulate pressure effectively.

Corticosteroids may also contribute to other metabolic changes that increase cardiovascular risk, including insulin resistance, weight gain, and dyslipidemia. These factors can compound the risk of developing hypertension, especially in individuals with existing health conditions. For patients requiring corticosteroids, it is important to use the lowest effective dose for the shortest duration possible. Monitoring blood pressure closely during treatment is essential for minimizing long-term harm.

4. Oral Contraceptives

Oral contraceptives are one of the most commonly used forms of birth control worldwide. Certain formulations containing synthetic estrogen and progestin have been linked to elevated blood pressure. The risk is particularly significant for women who are over the age of 35, overweight, smokers, or those with a personal or family history of hypertension.

Oral contraceptives may raise blood pressure by influencing the body's renin-angiotensin-aldosterone system, which helps regulate fluid balance and vascular tone. Estrogen can increase hepatic production of angiotensinogen, a precursor to angiotensin II, which causes blood vessels to constrict. This leads to increased vascular resistance and higher blood pressure. In addition, contraceptives can promote fluid retention and alter electrolyte balance, both of which contribute to increased blood volume and pressure.

A large-scale study published in *The New England Journal of Medicine* found that women who used oral contraceptives were more likely to develop hypertension, particularly with long-term use or higher-dose estrogen formulations (Chasan-Taber et al., 1996). The effects are often more pronounced in women with underlying metabolic imbalances or cardiovascular risk factors. Monitoring blood pressure regularly is important for women using hormonal birth control.

5. Antidepressants

Antidepressants are widely prescribed to treat conditions such as depression, anxiety, and chronic pain. Certain types have been associated with increased blood pressure, depression, and suicidal thoughts. Understanding which classes of antidepressants affect cardiovascular health is important for those managing or seeking to reverse hypertension. Some antidepressants, especially serotonin-norepinephrine reuptake inhibitors (SNRIs) such as venlafaxine and duloxetine, can raise blood pressure by increasing levels of norepinephrine. This neurotransmitter stimulates the sympathetic nervous system, leading to vasoconstriction and a rise in both systolic and diastolic pressure. A study published in *Psychosomatic Medicine* found that high doses of venlafaxine significantly increased blood pressure in patients, particularly among those already at risk for cardiovascular disease (Thase et al., 2005).

Tricyclic antidepressants, including amitriptyline and nortriptyline, can also elevate blood pressure by affecting both norepinephrine and serotonin levels. These medications may cause additional side effects such as weight gain and fluid retention, which further strain the cardiovascular system. Additionally, tricyclics may interact with antihypertensive medications, reducing their effectiveness and complicating blood pressure management.

Selective serotonin reuptake inhibitors (SSRIs) may contribute to changes in blood pressure in some individuals, particularly when combined with other medications or underlying hormonal imbalances. A review published in *CNS Drugs* noted that while SSRIs have minimal cardiovascular effects in most people, careful monitoring is still recommended for patients with hypertension (Roose, 2003). For individuals with both mood disorders and elevated blood pressure, non-pharmaceutical strategies such as exercise, meditation, sleep optimization, and dietary changes may be effective in improving mood while supporting blood pressure regulation.

6. Stimulants

Stimulant medications are often prescribed for conditions such as attention deficit hyperactivity disorder (ADHD), narcolepsy, and occasionally for weight loss or fatigue. These drugs are known to increase both heart rate and blood pressure. Individuals with hypertension or those at risk for cardiovascular disease should exercise caution when using stimulants, whether prescribed or recreational.

Stimulants such as amphetamine, dextroamphetamine, and methylphenidate work by increasing levels of dopamine and norepinephrine in the brain. These neurotransmitters activate the sympathetic nervous system, which raises heart rate and causes blood vessels to constrict. This response can result in a sustained elevation in both systolic and diastolic blood pressure. A study published in *The Journal of Clinical Psychiatry* found that stimulant use was associated with significant increases in blood pressure and heart rate, especially with higher doses or long-term use (Hammerness et al., 2009).

In addition to prescription medications, common over-the-counter stimulants include caffeine and certain ingredients found in energy drinks, pre-workout

253 of4inst

supplements, and weight loss products. These substances may further amplify cardiovascular strain, especially when used in combination with prescribed stimulants or consumed in large quantities.

For individuals already managing high blood pressure, stimulants may interfere with the effectiveness of antihypertensive medications. They may also increase the risk of complications such as arrhythmias, anxiety, insomnia, and vascular inflammation. Some patients with ADHD may benefit from non-stimulant treatment options. Careful monitoring of blood pressure is essential for anyone taking stimulant medications. It is also important to address underlying contributors to fatigue or inattention, such as poor sleep, nutrient deficiencies, chronic stress, or blood sugar imbalances, which may reduce or eliminate the need for stimulant use.

7. Immunosuppressive Medications

Immunosuppressive medications are used to prevent organ transplant rejection and to manage autoimmune diseases such as lupus, rheumatoid arthritis, and inflammatory bowel disease. These drugs can have significant side effects, including an increased risk of high blood pressure. The impact on blood pressure depends on the specific medication, dosage, duration of use, and the patient's overall health status.

One of the most common classes of immunosuppressants associated with elevated blood pressure is calcineurin inhibitors, including cyclosporine and tacrolimus. These medications affect kidney function by constricting the afferent arterioles in the kidneys, which reduces the filtration rate and promotes sodium and water retention. This leads to increased blood volume and vascular resistance. A study published in the *American Journal of Transplantation* found that up to 80 percent of kidney transplant recipients taking calcineurin inhibitors developed new or worsened hypertension within the first year of treatment (Midtvedt et al., 2003).

Other immunosuppressants, such as corticosteroids, which are often prescribed in combination with other drugs, can also contribute to elevated blood pressure through fluid retention, hormonal changes, and vascular sensitivity. The combined effect of multiple medications may compound cardiovascular stress and impair long-term blood pressure regulation.

In addition to their renal and vascular effects, some immunosuppressive drugs increase oxidative stress and reduce nitric oxide availability, both of which impair the ability of blood vessels to relax. These changes can lead to persistent vascular constriction and reduced responsiveness to antihypertensive therapy. For individuals taking immunosuppressants, regular monitoring of blood pressure and kidney function is critical. Adjusting the medication dosage, modifying the treatment plan, or implementing targeted lifestyle changes may help manage or prevent hypertension. Nutrient-rich diets, adequate hydration, and stress-reduction techniques may also support cardiovascular and immune health without compromising the primary treatment goals.

8. Chemotherapy and Targeted Cancer Therapies

Chemotherapy and targeted cancer therapies can come with significant side effects, including the development or worsening of high blood pressure. As cancer therapies become more common, understanding their cardiovascular impact has become increasingly important, especially for long-term health and recovery. Certain chemotherapy agents, such as cisplatin and cyclophosphamide, can cause vascular damage, promote oxidative stress, and impair kidney function. These effects can lead to sodium and water retention, increased vascular resistance, and ultimately, elevated blood pressure. Chemotherapy can also trigger inflammation and disrupt hormonal balance, which further interferes with the body's ability to regulate blood pressure effectively.

Targeted therapies, including vascular endothelial growth factor (VEGF) inhibitors such as bevacizumab, sorafenib, and sunitinib, have a particularly strong association with hypertension. These medications are designed to block the growth of new blood vessels in tumors, but they also reduce nitric oxide production and increase vascular stiffness. A meta-analysis published in *The Lancet Oncology* found that VEGF inhibitors significantly increase the risk of both mild and severe hypertension, with incidence rates exceeding 30 percent in some studies (Choueiri et al., 2010).

The cardiovascular side effects of these therapies may appear early in treatment or emerge gradually over time. If left unmanaged, therapy-induced hypertension can lead to complications such as heart failure, kidney damage, and increased risk of stroke. These risks are amplified in patients who already have elevated blood pressure or other underlying cardiovascular conditions.

Monitoring blood pressure regularly during cancer treatment is essential. Supportive strategies, including a low-sodium anti-inflammatory diet, stress management, and kidney support, can help reduce the cardiovascular burden while allowing patients to continue necessary cancer therapies.

Conclusion

Medication-induced hypertension is an important clinical consideration, especially for patients with existing cardiovascular risk factors or diagnosed hypertension. Healthcare providers and patients should monitor blood pressure closely when initiating or adjusting medications known to impact cardiovascular health. Awareness and proactive management, including medication adjustments or lifestyle interventions, can significantly reduce the risk of drug-induced hypertension.

Medicinal Teas

Tea has been consumed for centuries not only for its soothing properties but also for its powerful medicinal effects. Certain herbal and non-herbal teas contain bioactive compounds that have been shown to support cardiovascular health by lowering blood pressure naturally. This chapter explores the most effective blood pressure-lowering teas, the active compounds involved, and the supporting scientific evidence. Herbal teas have been used for centuries to support cardiovascular health. Several types of teas have demonstrated blood pressure-lowering effects due to their anti-inflammatory, antioxidant, and vasorelaxant properties. The following teas are among the most well-researched for their role in managing hypertension.

Hibiscus Tea:

Hibiscus tea, made from the dried petals of the *Hibiscus sabdariffa* flower, is one of the most extensively studied herbal teas for blood pressure control. It contains anthocyanins and other polyphenolic compounds that support endothelial function and reduce arterial stiffness. A randomized controlled trial published in the *Journal of Nutrition* found that drinking three cups of hibiscus tea daily for six weeks led to significant reductions in systolic blood pressure, with average reductions of up to 7.2 mm Hg in prehypertensive and mildly hypertensive adults (McKay et al., 2010). Another meta-analysis of five clinical trials confirmed that hibiscus tea significantly lowers both systolic and diastolic blood pressure in a dose-dependent manner (Serban et al., 2015). Its effects are often comparable to standard antihypertensive medications, especially when combined with dietary changes.

Green Tea:

Green tea is rich in catechins, particularly epigallocatechin gallate (EGCG), which has powerful antioxidant and vasodilatory effects. Regular consumption is associated with improved endothelial function, reduced oxidative stress, and decreased vascular resistance. A meta-analysis of 13 randomized controlled trials found that green tea consumption resulted in statistically significant reductions in both systolic and diastolic blood pressure, particularly when consumed consistently for longer than 12 weeks (Peng et al., 2014). Additional findings from a separate meta-analysis suggested that green tea may also reduce blood pressure variability, which is an important factor in cardiovascular risk (Khalesi et al., 2014).

Oolong Tea:

Oolong tea is a semi-fermented tea that contains a blend of catechins and theaflavins known for their antioxidant and lipid-lowering effects. It has demonstrated potential for reducing blood pressure in both observational and clinical research. A population-based study conducted in Taiwan involving over 1,500 participants found that those who drank green or oolong tea daily for at least one year had a 46 percent lower risk of developing hypertension compared to non-tea drinkers (Yang et al., 2004). Another study in China confirmed similar findings, showing that habitual oolong tea consumption was associated with reduced systolic blood pressure and a lower risk of cardiovascular events (Zhang et al., 2011).

Rooibos Tea:

Rooibos, or *Aspalathus linearis*, is a naturally caffeine-free tea native to South Africa. It is rich in unique polyphenols such as aspalathin and nothofagin, which demonstrate anti-inflammatory, antioxidant, and vasorelaxant properties. A pilot study published in the *Journal of Ethnopharmacology* showed that rooibos extract improved vascular tone and reduced oxidative stress in adults with increased cardiovascular risk (Persson et al., 2010). Although fewer clinical trials exist compared to other teas, emerging evidence suggests that rooibos may help improve endothelial function and support blood pressure regulation, particularly when consumed regularly.

Chamomile Tea:

Chamomile is traditionally known for its calming effects, but it also contains flavonoids and apigenin, which may have mild antihypertensive properties. By promoting relaxation and reducing sympathetic nervous system activity, chamomile may help lower stress-induced spikes in blood pressure. A study conducted at the University of Pennsylvania showed that chamomile extract significantly reduced anxiety symptoms in individuals with generalized anxiety disorder, which may indirectly improve cardiovascular outcomes (Amsterdam et al., 2009). Additional evidence from small human trials and animal studies suggests that chamomile may reduce systolic blood pressure through parasympathetic nervous system activation and smooth muscle relaxation.

Lavender and Lemon Balm Tea:

Lavender and lemon balm are herbs known for their ability to reduce anxiety and promote calmness. These herbs act on the central nervous system to reduce stress hormone levels, which can contribute to blood pressure regulation. A clinical trial published in *Phytomedicine* showed that lemon balm extract significantly reduced stress-related blood pressure elevations and improved autonomic nervous system balance (Kennedy et al., 2004). Lavender has shown similar effects in small human trials, helping to modulate cortisol and promote relaxation, both of which contribute to healthier blood pressure levels.

Conclusion

Teas can be a gentle yet effective natural intervention for managing high blood pressure. Regular consumption of hibiscus, green, oolong, rooibos, chamomile, and lemon balm tea, when combined with a healthy lifestyle, may offer measurable improvements in cardiovascular health. Choosing organic, additive-free teas and avoiding added sugars or artificial flavors is essential to maximize health benefits.

Vitamin, Mineral, and Hormonal Imbalances

The Role of Vitamin, Mineral, and Hormonal Deficiencies in High Blood Pressure

High blood pressure, or hypertension, is a multifactorial condition influenced not only by lifestyle and genetics but also by nutritional and hormonal imbalances. Research has identified several vitamin, mineral, and hormone deficiencies that may contribute to elevated blood pressure. Because individual biochemical needs vary, personalized lab testing is essential for identifying deficiencies and guiding effective supplementation. Managing high blood pressure naturally requires a tailored approach that targets these underlying imbalances.

From my clinical experience, I have observed that most individuals with hypertension have between **four to eight vitamin and mineral deficiencies** that significantly impact their blood pressure. When these deficiencies are addressed with the proper form and dosage of supplements, blood pressure often returns to a normal range. Chronic hypertension is rarely the result of a single cause. Micronutrient deficiencies and hormonal imbalances often play a central role in the development and persistence of elevated blood pressure. Identifying and correcting these imbalances through laboratory testing and targeted supplementation may significantly improve vascular function and reduce cardiovascular risk.

Vitamin D Deficiency:

Vitamin D plays a critical role in modulating the renin-angiotensin system, reducing inflammation, and supporting endothelial function. Low serum levels are associated with increased arterial stiffness, vascular dysfunction, and elevated systolic and diastolic pressure. A meta-analysis by Kunutsor et al. (2013) concluded that individuals with low vitamin D levels had a significantly higher risk of developing hypertension. Another systematic review by Beveridge et al. (2015) confirmed that vitamin D supplementation can lead to modest but clinically meaningful reductions in blood pressure, particularly in individuals with baseline deficiency. Optimal dosing requires lab-guided monitoring, as excessive vitamin D may lead to hypercalcemia, kidney strain, and increased cardiovascular risk.

Magnesium Deficiency:

Magnesium supports vascular tone, smooth muscle relaxation, and intracellular calcium regulation. Deficiency has been linked to increased sympathetic nervous system activity and impaired endothelial function. A meta-analysis of 34 clinical trials by Zhang et al. (2016) found that magnesium supplementation significantly reduced systolic and diastolic blood pressure, especially in individuals with hypertension or low baseline magnesium levels. An earlier study by Rosanoff et al. (2012) confirmed that daily magnesium intake was associated with improved blood pressure regulation. Excessive intake may cause gastrointestinal symptoms, confusion, cardiac arrest, and kidney dysfunction, emphasizing the need for personalized dosing.

Vitamin B2 (Riboflavin) Deficiency:

Riboflavin acts as a coenzyme in redox reactions and is essential for homocysteine metabolism. Elevated homocysteine contributes to oxidative stress and endothelial dysfunction. A study by Wilson et al. (2012) demonstrated that riboflavin supplementation significantly lowered blood pressure in individuals with the MTHFR 677TT genotype, a variant associated with impaired folate metabolism and increased cardiovascular risk. This genetic subgroup may benefit significantly from targeted riboflavin support as part of a comprehensive cardiovascular care plan.

Vitamin B12 (Cobalamin) Deficiency:

Vitamin B12 is essential for red blood cell formation, nervous system function, and methylation. Deficiency leads to elevated homocysteine and oxidative stress, which can impair nitric oxide production and vascular elasticity. A study by Herrmann et al. (2007) found that low B12 levels were correlated with increased arterial stiffness and blood pressure. Additional research by den Elzen et al. (2008) confirmed that vitamin B12 deficiency is common in older adults with hypertension and contributes to poor vascular outcomes. Regular monitoring of B12, homocysteine, and methylmalonic acid is recommended to guide treatment. Excessive intake may cause numbness, burning sensations, and itching, emphasizing the need for personalized dosing.

Vitamin B6 (Pyridoxine) Deficiency:

Vitamin B6 is involved in amino acid metabolism, neurotransmitter synthesis, and homocysteine regulation. Deficiency may increase vascular inflammation and interfere with nitric oxide signaling. A study by Verhoef et al. (2002) reported that vitamin B6 deficiency was associated with higher blood pressure and cardiovascular risk. Supplementation has been shown to lower homocysteine levels and may support improved endothelial function and vascular tone. Excessive intake of vitamin B6 may lead to nerve damage, numbness, and tingling in the hands and feet, highlighting the importance of personalized dosing.

Folate (Vitamin B9) Deficiency:

Folate plays a key role in DNA synthesis and the methylation cycle. Low intake or poor absorption can raise homocysteine levels, damaging the endothelium and increasing the risk of hypertension. A prospective study by Forman et al. (2005) involving over 150,000 women found that higher folate intake was associated with a significantly lower risk of developing high blood pressure. Folate supplementation may be especially beneficial for individuals with MTHFR polymorphisms and those consuming diets low in leafy greens or legumes. Excessive intake of vitamin B9 may mask vitamin B12 deficiency and contribute to neurological damage, underscoring the importance of personalized dosing.

Coenzyme Q10 (CoQ10) Deficiency:

CoQ10 is a fat-soluble antioxidant that supports mitochondrial energy production and protects cells from oxidative damage. It also helps maintain nitric oxide levels and vascular elasticity. A meta-analysis by Rosenfeldt et al. (2007) found that CoQ10 supplementation reduced systolic blood pressure by an average of 11 mm Hg and diastolic pressure by 7 mm Hg in patients with hypertension. Another review by Ho et al. (2016) confirmed that CoQ10 improves endothelial function and may benefit patients with resistant hypertension or statin-induced CoQ10 depletion.

Iron Deficiency:

Iron is essential for hemoglobin production and oxygen delivery. Iron deficiency anemia may trigger hypoxia and stimulate the renin-angiotensin system, leading to compensatory increases in blood pressure. A study by Zacharski et al. (2000) showed that correcting iron deficiency in women improved cardiovascular markers and reduced blood pressure, particularly in those with fatigue or heavy menstrual cycles. However, excessive iron supplementation can promote oxidative stress, joint pain, liver dysfunction, and heart failure, so individualized dosing is critical.

Zinc Deficiency:

Zinc supports antioxidant defense, hormone regulation, and immune function. Deficiency impairs endothelial repair, promotes oxidative damage, and disrupts vascular tone. A study by Song et al. (2009) demonstrated that zinc supplementation reduced systolic blood pressure in hypertensive individuals with low baseline zinc levels. Other research has shown that zinc deficiency may exacerbate inflammation and contribute to vascular dysfunction. Supplementation should be carefully monitored, as excessive zinc can lead to copper depletion and hormonal imbalances.

Potassium Deficiency:

Potassium is a vital mineral that plays a central role in regulating blood pressure by balancing sodium levels, supporting kidney function, and maintaining vascular tone. A deficiency in potassium disrupts this balance, contributing to fluid retention, increased vascular resistance, and elevated blood pressure. The modern diet, which is often high in processed foods and low in fresh fruits and vegetables, typically provides far less potassium than needed for optimal cardiovascular health. This imbalance between high sodium intake and low potassium intake creates a biochemical environment that promotes hypertension and increases the risk of stroke and cardiovascular disease.

Several large-scale studies have confirmed the inverse relationship between potassium intake and blood pressure. The INTERSALT study, which included over 10,000 participants from 32 countries, found that higher urinary potassium excretion, a marker of greater dietary potassium intake, was associated with lower systolic and diastolic blood pressure. Similarly, a meta-analysis published in *BMJ* concluded that potassium supplementation significantly reduced both systolic and diastolic blood pressure, particularly in individuals with hypertension and those consuming high amounts of sodium. These findings suggest that correcting potassium deficiency through diet or supplementation is a safe and effective strategy for lowering blood pressure.

Potassium-rich foods such as avocados, leafy greens, sweet potatoes, bananas, and beans should be emphasized in any blood pressure-lowering dietary plan. In cases where dietary intake is insufficient or when blood testing reveals a deficiency, targeted potassium supplementation may be necessary. However, supplementation should be monitored closely by a healthcare provider, especially in individuals with kidney disease or those taking medications that affect potassium balance. Excessive potassium intake, particularly from supplements, can lead to hyperkalemia, a condition marked by dangerously high potassium levels in the blood. Symptoms of hyperkalemia include muscle weakness, irregular heartbeat, and in severe cases, cardiac arrest. Potassium overload may also cause kidney dysfunction and impair neuromuscular function. For this reason, laboratory testing of serum potassium and kidney function is essential before initiating supplementation. Proper assessment ensures that potassium levels are corrected safely and effectively without placing additional strain on vital organs.

Estrogen and Progesterone Imbalances:

Sex hormones influence blood pressure regulation through their effects on nitric oxide production, vascular reactivity, and sodium handling. Estrogen helps maintain endothelial health, while progesterone has natural diuretic properties and supports vascular relaxation. A review by Reckelhoff (2001) found that hormonal imbalances, especially in postmenopausal women, contribute to increased risk of hypertension. Estrogen dominance or progesterone deficiency may lead to fluid retention and increased vascular tension. Hormone testing and functional support may help restore hormonal balance and improve blood pressure control.

Thyroid Hormone Imbalances:

Thyroid hormones regulate metabolism, heart rate, and vascular resistance. Hypothyroidism, including subclinical cases, is associated with increased diastolic blood pressure and systemic vascular resistance. A study by Udovcic et al. (2017) confirmed that individuals with subclinical hypothyroidism are more likely to experience elevated blood pressure, especially older adults. Testing thyroid-stimulating hormone (TSH), free T3, and free T4 is essential when evaluating unexplained or treatment-resistant hypertension.

Cortisol Dysregulation (Adrenal Imbalance)

Cortisol, the body's primary stress hormone, influences blood pressure by regulating sodium retention, vascular tone, and inflammatory pathways. Chronic stress or adrenal dysregulation can lead to sustained elevation in cortisol levels and contribute to resistant hypertension. A review by Whitworth et al. (2005) highlighted the strong link between cortisol excess and elevated blood pressure. Addressing adrenal health through stress management, adaptogenic herbs, and functional testing may be critical for individuals with stress-related hypertension.

Conclusion

Identifying and correcting vitamin, mineral, and hormonal deficiencies through lab testing is a foundational strategy for reversing high blood pressure naturally. While generalized supplementation may offer short term benefits, a personalized approach ensures optimal dosing and avoids potential side effects. Collaborating with a clinical nutritionist is essential for creating a targeted, effective plan.

Correcting nutrient deficiencies such as vitamin D, magnesium, CoQ10, and B complex vitamins can reduce vascular inflammation, enhance endothelial function, and support healthy blood pressure regulation. Clinically, individuals with hypertension often present with multiple nutrient deficiencies. In my experience treating patients with chronic diseases, most individuals with **hypertension exhibit at least four to eight deficiencies**. Addressing these through diet and targeted supplementation has been a game changer in helping patients lower blood pressure and improve cardiovascular health. However, supplementation must be approached with precision and guided by professional oversight. Partnering with a clinical nutritionist is essential for accurately identifying deficiencies and determining appropriate dosing for each individual.

Optimizing hormone levels, especially thyroid and sex hormones, is equally important for long term blood pressure stability and cardiovascular health. Taking an integrative approach that combines diagnostic testing, targeted supplementation, dietary adjustments, and stress management empowers individuals to regain control over their health. Addressing root causes, not just symptoms, leads to more sustainable outcomes in the prevention and reversal of hypertension.

Exercise

Exercise for Lowering Blood Pressure

Regular physical activity is one of the most effective natural strategies for reducing high blood pressure (hypertension). Engaging in consistent exercise helps improve heart health, reduce stress levels, enhance vascular function, and support hormonal balance, all of which contribute to lowering blood pressure. The American Heart Association recommends at least 150 minutes of moderate-intensity aerobic exercise per week for optimal cardiovascular health (Pescatello et al., 2015).

Benefits of Exercise for Blood Pressure:

1. **Improved Vascular Function**: Exercise enhances endothelial function, which is crucial for maintaining flexible and healthy blood vessels. This improvement reduces peripheral resistance and allows blood to flow more freely, helping to lower blood pressure (Green et al., 2004).
2. **Weight Management**: Physical activity helps maintain a healthy body weight, and even modest weight loss can lead to meaningful reductions in blood pressure (Stevens et al., 2001).
3. **Stress Reduction**: Exercise is a powerful stress reliever. It decreases cortisol levels and increases endorphin production, which improves mood and reduces anxiety, a known contributor to elevated blood pressure (Paluska & Schwenk, 2000).
4. **Enhanced Insulin Sensitivity**: Regular movement improves the body's sensitivity to insulin and helps regulate blood sugar levels, which can indirectly lower blood pressure (Ross et al., 2000).
5. **Lower Resting Heart Rate**: Cardiovascular conditioning through exercise lowers resting heart rate and cardiac workload, promoting better overall cardiovascular function.

Types of Exercises That Help Lower Blood Pressure

Several types of exercise have been shown to significantly reduce blood pressure, many of which can be done at home without special equipment:

1. Aerobic Exercise

- **Examples**: Brisk walking, jogging in place, dancing, stair climbing, cycling on a stationary bike
- **Benefits**: Lowers both systolic and diastolic blood pressure by improving heart efficiency and reducing vascular resistance (Cornelissen & Fagard, 2005).
- **At-Home Tip**: Aim for 30 minutes of brisk walking or dancing daily.

2. Resistance Training

- **Examples**: Bodyweight exercises (push-ups, squats, lunges), resistance bands
- **Benefits**: Increases lean muscle mass, improves insulin sensitivity, and contributes to blood pressure reduction (MacDonald et al., 2016).
- **At-Home Tip**: Perform 2–3 sets of 10–15 reps of major muscle group exercises, 2–3 times per week.

3. Isometric Exercises

- **Examples**: Wall sits, plank holds, handgrip exercises
- **Benefits**: Emerging evidence shows isometric exercises can lead to significant reductions in resting blood pressure, especially systolic pressure (Inder et al., 2016).
- **At-Home Tip**: Try 2-minute wall sits or handgrip squeezes several times a week.

4. Mind-Body Exercises

- **Examples**: Yoga, tai chi, deep breathing exercises
- **Benefits**: Promote relaxation, reduce cortisol levels, and improve heart rate variability, all of which are beneficial for lowering blood pressure (Cui et al., 2016).
- **At-Home Tip**: Incorporate 10–20 minutes of gentle yoga or guided breathing exercises daily.

A Simple Way to Lower Blood Pressure and Blood Sugar While You Sit

Using an under-desk bike or elliptical is a simple yet effective way to stay active while watching TV or working at your computer. These compact machines allow you to pedal gently while seated, making it easy to add movement into your daily routine without interrupting your activities. Whether you're catching up on emails, watching your favorite show, or reading on your tablet, you can be improving your health at the same time.

Regular use of an under-desk bike or elliptical can help lower both blood pressure and blood sugar levels. Even light physical activity promotes better circulation, improves insulin sensitivity, and supports cardiovascular health. For people with a sedentary lifestyle or limited mobility, this can be a game-changer for managing chronic health issues naturally and safely.

I personally recommend this type of exercise for older adults who may be fragile or unable to walk for long periods. It's also ideal for those living in areas where weather conditions limit outdoor activity. The machine is easy to store and use, requiring little space and no complicated setup. Start with 5–10 minutes a day and gradually build up to 30–45 minutes. It offers a low-impact, convenient way to stay active and support your overall wellness.

Exercise Safety and Considerations

- Start gradually and consult with a healthcare provider if you have any underlying conditions.
- Maintain hydration and proper form to avoid injury.
- Combine different types of exercise for maximum cardiovascular and stress-reducing benefits.

Conclusion

Exercise is a powerful, low-cost, and natural method for lowering blood pressure. By incorporating various forms of aerobic, resistance, isometric, and mind-body exercises into your daily routine, you can experience improved cardiovascular health, reduced stress levels, and better overall well-being. Making exercise a consistent part of your lifestyle is an essential step in managing and reversing high blood pressure.

Stress Management

The Link Between Stress and High Blood Pressure

Stress is widely recognized as a significant contributing factor to high blood pressure, also known as hypertension. Research indicates that both acute and chronic stress can substantially influence blood pressure levels. Approximately 75% of adults report stress as a major contributor to their high blood pressure episodes (American Heart Association, 2022). Studies have demonstrated that frequent fluctuations in stress levels, rather than consistent stress, may trigger acute elevations in blood pressure. A notable study published in the journal *Hypertension* found that individuals experiencing daily stressors exhibited significant spikes in blood pressure, particularly when transitioning from high-stress periods to relaxation. This illustrates the "let-down effect" (Steptoe & Kivimäki, 2013).

Physiological Mechanisms Linking Stress to Hypertension

The connection between stress and hypertension primarily involves activation of the hypothalamic-pituitary-adrenal (HPA) axis and the sympathetic nervous system. When confronted with stress, the body releases stress hormones, particularly cortisol and adrenaline. These hormones lead to increased heart rate, blood vessel constriction, and elevated blood pressure levels (Chrousos, 2009). Chronic activation of the HPA axis can cause persistent elevations in cortisol levels, contributing to sustained blood pressure increases and promoting inflammation and vascular damage (Whitworth et al., 2005). Moreover, prolonged stress can result in endothelial dysfunction, reducing blood vessels' capacity to dilate properly and further exacerbating hypertension (Rozanski et al., 2005).

Stress and Reduced Effectiveness of Hypertension Treatments

Stress can also negatively impact the effectiveness of antihypertensive treatments. Studies indicate that individuals under significant stress often experience less effective control of blood pressure through medications and lifestyle changes (Rozanski et al., 2005). Managing stress effectively is, therefore, crucial in improving treatment outcomes and reducing hypertension-related complications.

Stress, Trauma, and Hypertension

Chronic stress is one of the most overlooked but powerful contributors to high blood pressure. When the body perceives a threat, whether physical or emotional, it activates the sympathetic nervous system, triggering the release of stress hormones such as cortisol and adrenaline. These hormones increase heart rate, constrict blood vessels, and elevate blood pressure to prepare the body for immediate action. While this response is adaptive in the short term, prolonged activation, which is common in individuals facing chronic life stress, financial strain, relationship challenges, or emotional trauma, can lead to sustained hypertension and cardiovascular strain.

Unresolved trauma, including post-traumatic stress disorder (PTSD), plays a significant role in this process. The body of someone with PTSD often remains in a state of hypervigilance and physiological arousal long after the threat has passed. Studies have shown that individuals with PTSD are significantly more likely to develop hypertension and cardiovascular disease. The repeated activation of stress pathways disrupts hormonal balance, impairs endothelial function, and contributes to systemic inflammation, all of which raise blood pressure over time.

Addressing trauma and emotional stress is essential for reversing high blood pressure at its root. Stress-reduction strategies such as deep breathing, meditation, exercise, and counseling can help regulate the nervous system and reduce sympathetic activity. However, when hypertension is linked to unresolved trauma, chronic anxiety, or depression, these tools may not be enough on their own. Depression, in particular, is a significant psychological factor that contributes to elevated blood pressure. It is often accompanied by disrupted sleep, low energy, poor dietary habits, and increased inflammation, all of which contribute to heightened cardiovascular risk. Depression also alters the brain's stress response by overactivating the hypothalamic pituitary adrenal (HPA) axis and increasing cortisol levels, which can raise heart rate, impair vascular function, and elevate blood pressure over time.

Furthermore, individuals with depression often struggle to maintain healthy routines such as regular physical activity, balanced nutrition, and consistent medication use, making blood pressure control more difficult. For those dealing with anxiety, depression, or the lasting effects of trauma, it is important to treat the underlying mental and emotional imbalances. My book *Beating Anxiety and Depression* offers a comprehensive, natural approach to healing these root causes. By restoring mental and emotional balance, the body is better able to regulate blood pressure and achieve long-term cardiovascular health.

Effects of Stress on Different Biological Systems

Scientific research consistently underscores stress's broad physiological impacts, contributing to multiple health conditions:

- **Cardiovascular Effects**: Chronic stress can lead to increased heart rate, sustained high blood pressure, atherosclerosis, and increased risks of heart attack and stroke.
- **Metabolic Effects**: Stress elevates blood glucose levels, increasing the risk of type 2 diabetes and metabolic syndrome.
- **Gastrointestinal Effects**: Stress disrupts digestive processes, leading to conditions such as acid reflux, stomach ulcers, constipation, or diarrhea.
- **Musculoskeletal Effects**: Chronic stress causes muscle tension and chronic pain, including headaches, back pain, and neck stiffness.
- **Reproductive Effects**: Stress can disrupt hormonal balances, impacting testosterone levels in men and menstrual regularity in women.
- **Immune System Effects**: Persistent stress suppresses immune system function, making the body more susceptible to infections.
- **Neurological and Psychological Effects**: Stress contributes to anxiety, depression, cognitive impairment, and sleep disorders.

Mechanisms of Muscle Tension Due to Stress

- **Fight-or-Flight Response**: Stress triggers the body's natural "fight-or-flight" mechanism, causing muscles to tighten in preparation for physical action.
- **Cortisol Release**: Elevated cortisol levels from stress induce prolonged muscle tension.
- **Neuromuscular Activation**: Chronic stress maintains muscles in a semi-contracted state, causing discomfort and stiffness.

Consequences of Chronic Muscle Tension

- **Pain and Discomfort**: Sustained muscle tension results in chronic pain, headaches, and overall physical discomfort.
- **Reduced Mobility**: Chronic muscle tension can impair joint mobility and posture, increasing injury risk.
- **Trigger Points and Fibrotic Tissue**: Persistent muscle tension contributes to trigger points and fibrotic tissues, exacerbating musculoskeletal pain.
- **Fatigue**: Constantly tense muscles consume significant energy, causing general fatigue and reduced physical performance.

Strategies for Managing Stress

Managing stress is essential for controlling blood pressure and enhancing overall health. Consider incorporating these evidence-based approaches:

- **Identify Stressors**: Maintain a stress journal to pinpoint sources and patterns.
- **Regular Physical Activity**: Exercise consistently to release endorphins and reduce stress hormones.
- **Mindfulness and Meditation**: Practice mindfulness, deep breathing exercises, and meditation to decrease stress responses.
- **Time Management**: Prioritize tasks effectively, break projects into manageable steps, and establish clear boundaries.
- **Healthy Lifestyle Choices**: Maintain proper nutrition, hydration, and adequate sleep.
- **Social Support**: Foster strong social connections and openly discuss stressors with trusted individuals.

By implementing these stress reduction strategies, individuals can significantly lower their blood pressure and improve cardiovascular health.

Simple Breathing Meditation for Calm and Clarity

One of the easiest and most effective mindfulness practices is breathing meditation. By focusing on your breath, you train your mind to stay present and let go of distractions.

1. Basic Breathing Meditation (5 Minutes)

Step 1: Find a quiet, comfortable space to sit. Keep your spine straight but relaxed.
Step 2: Close your eyes and bring your attention to your breath.
Step 3: Breathe in slowly through your nose, feeling your belly expand.
Step 4: Exhale gently through your mouth, feeling tension leave your body.
Step 5: If your mind wanders, gently bring it back to the breath.
   Tip: Set a timer for 5 minutes and gradually increase to 10–15 minutes over time.

2. The 4-7-8 Relaxation Breath (For Stress Relief)

A powerful technique for calming the nervous system.
Step 1: Inhale deeply through your nose for 4 seconds.
Step 2: Hold your breath for 7 seconds.
Step 3: Slowly exhale through your mouth for 8 seconds.
Step 4: Repeat for 4 rounds.
✅ Best for: Reducing stress, improving sleep, calming anxiety.

3. Box Breathing (For Focus and Clarity)

A technique used by Navy SEALs to enhance concentration under pressure.
Step 1: Inhale for 4 seconds.
Step 2: Hold the breath for 4 seconds.
Step 3: Exhale for 4 seconds.
Step 4: Hold again for 4 seconds.
Step 5: Repeat for 5 minutes.
✅ Best for: Enhancing focus, relieving anxiety, preparing for high-stress situations.

4. Mindful Walking (For Mental Clarity)

Instead of walking on autopilot, turn it into a grounding mindfulness practice.
Step 1: Walk slowly and intentionally, feeling the movement of your feet.
Step 2: Focus on the sensation of your breath, the wind, and the ground beneath you.

Step 3: Observe your surroundings without judgment.

Step 4: If your mind wanders, gently bring it back to the present.

✅ Best for: Reducing stress, clearing the mind, breaking up long work sessions.

5. Body Scan Meditation (For Deep Relaxation)

Helps release physical tension and stress stored in the body.

Step 1: Lie down in a comfortable position.

Step 2: Close your eyes and take a deep breath.

Step 3: Slowly bring your attention to each body part, starting from your feet and moving upwards.

Step 4: Notice any tension or discomfort, and consciously relax that area.

Step 5: Finish by taking three deep breaths and slowly opening your eyes.

✅ Best for: Relaxation, reducing muscle tension, preparing for sleep.

How to Make Mindfulness a Daily Habit

◆ Start small: Just 5 minutes a day can make a difference.

◆ Pair it with daily routines: Meditate after waking up or before bedtime.

◆ Use reminders: Set phone alerts or place sticky notes as mindfulness cues.

◆ Be patient: Mindfulness is a skill that improves with practice.

Conclusion

Managing stress is an essential part of reducing hypertension. Chronic stress activates the body's fight or flight response, leading to inflammation, muscle tension, hormonal disruption, and neurological overstimulation key factors that can trigger or worsen hypertension. While this chapter provides tools for managing everyday stress, it is important to recognize that deeper emotional struggles such as anxiety, depression, and post-traumatic stress disorder (PTSD) require more comprehensive support.

If you are dealing with chronic anxiety, emotional overwhelm, or unresolved trauma, I encourage you to explore my companion book **Beating Anxiety and Depression**: *14 Natural Secrets to a Happier Life*. This book offers a step-by-step natural approach to emotional healing backed by research and clinical experience. It addresses the biological, psychological, and lifestyle factors that contribute to mental health struggles and provides actionable strategies to restore emotional balance.

Due to the complexity of mental health conditions, it is difficult to do justice to this topic in just one chapter. That is why *Beating Anxiety and Depression* was created as a complete resource for those seeking long-term relief from anxiety, depression, and PTSD. If emotional stress plays a role in your hypertension or if you are simply looking to improve your mental well-being, this book is a powerful next step on your healing journey.

BEATING ANXIETY & DEPRESSION

BONUS VIDEOS

14 NATURAL SECRETS TO A HAPPIER LIFE

- Conquer Anxiety & Depression Naturally
- Heal the Root Causes & Reclaim Your Life
- Created by a Doctor Who Conquered PTSD & Depression
- Science-Based Strategies for Lasting Change

Dr. Joseph Jacobs, DPT, ACN

Behavior Modification

Behavior Modification for Lowering Blood Pressure

Behavior modification plays a foundational role in managing and reversing high blood pressure. Unlike quick fixes or medications that only address symptoms, behavior change tackles the root causes of hypertension by transforming daily habits and long-term lifestyle patterns. The following seven elements of behavior modification are supported by research and have been shown to significantly reduce blood pressure when consistently implemented.

1. Dietary Changes

Following the ASTR Diet is a powerful and natural approach to lowering high blood pressure by addressing its root causes. Detailed in my book *Eat to Heal*, the ASTR Diet was developed after overcoming chronic fatigue, pain, and migraines. This diet focuses on four key principles: anti-inflammatory, sustainable, toxin free, and restorative. By eliminating inflammatory foods and emphasizing nutrient-dense whole foods, such as leafy greens, healthy fats, gluten free grains, and antioxidant-rich fruits, the ASTR Diet helps reduce systemic inflammation and support healthy blood vessel function.

It also avoids common triggers such as refined carbohydrates, processed meats, and artificial additives that can contribute to vascular damage and hormonal imbalances. Many individuals with hypertension also experience multiple nutrient deficiencies, and the ASTR Diet naturally replenishes vital nutrients such as magnesium, potassium, and vitamin D. By restoring cellular balance and optimizing metabolic health, the ASTR Diet provides a science-backed and holistic pathway to achieving and maintaining healthy blood pressure.

2. Regular Physical Activity

Exercise improves cardiovascular function, reduces stress hormones, and promotes weight management. Even moderate-intensity activity such as walking, swimming, or home-based aerobic workouts can reduce systolic blood pressure by 4–9 mm Hg (Cornelissen & Fagard, 2005). Consistency is critical, so aim for at least 150 minutes of moderate activity per week.

3. Stress Reduction

Chronic stress contributes to hormonal imbalances, inflammation, and vascular dysfunction. Mindfulness practices, deep breathing, progressive muscle relaxation, and guided meditation are all effective ways to lower stress and blood pressure. One meta-analysis found that stress management interventions significantly reduced both systolic and diastolic blood pressure (Blumenthal et al., 2010).

4. Improving Sleep Quality

Sleep is a powerful regulator of blood pressure. Poor sleep quality and sleep deprivation are associated with increased sympathetic nervous system activity and elevated blood pressure. Prioritizing 7–9 hours of restful sleep, maintaining a consistent sleep schedule, and minimizing screen time before bed can support cardiovascular health (Palagini et al., 2013).

5. Limiting Alcohol and Quitting Smoking

Both alcohol and tobacco have strong associations with elevated blood pressure and increased cardiovascular risk. Cutting back on alcohol and quitting smoking can significantly reduce blood pressure and improve overall health outcomes (Virdis et al., 2010).

6. Accountability and Social Support

People are more successful at making lasting lifestyle changes when they have accountability and support. Joining a wellness group, working with a health coach, or engaging in supportive social networks can reinforce behavior change and improve adherence. Studies show that peer support is positively correlated with long-term hypertension control (Heisler et al., 2010).

7. Tracking Progress and Setting Goals

Self-monitoring behaviors such as tracking blood pressure, dietary intake, activity levels, and sleep help individuals stay informed and motivated. Setting small, achievable goals and celebrating progress reinforces positive habits and increases the likelihood of sustained change.

8. Nutrient Deficiencies and Hypertension

Identifying and addressing vitamin and mineral deficiencies is a crucial yet often overlooked component of managing hypertension. In my clinical experience, patients with high blood pressure typically present with **four to eight nutrient deficiencies**, many of which directly affect vascular function, inflammation, and fluid balance. Common deficiencies include magnesium, potassium, iron, vitamin D, and B-complex vitamins. These nutrients play vital roles in regulating blood pressure. When these deficiencies go unaddressed, they can silently perpetuate hypertension, even in patients who are exercising and eating relatively well.

It is essential to work with a qualified clinical nutritionist to accurately assess and correct these imbalances. Supplementation must be tailored to the individual. Improper dosing, can lead to suboptimal outcomes or adverse effects. A clinical nutritionist can order targeted lab testing, interpret the results within the context of the patient's overall health, and design a personalized nutrition plan that includes appropriate dietary adjustments and evidence-based supplementation. Without professional guidance, many individuals unknowingly continue to live with nutrient deficiencies that fuel hypertension, despite making efforts to improve their lifestyle. Addressing these hidden deficiencies under expert supervision can be a game-changing step toward naturally lowering blood pressure and reducing long-term cardiovascular risk.

Conclusion

Long-term blood pressure reduction requires more than temporary solutions. Behavior modification empowers individuals to take control of their health by making intentional, sustainable changes to their daily habits. By addressing multiple lifestyle factors and staying consistent, individuals can not only lower their blood pressure but also prevent future complications and improve their overall quality of life.

Conclusion

Your Healing Starts Now

You've reached the final chapter of this book, but in many ways, this is just the beginning. High blood pressure is not simply a diagnosis to manage. It is a signal that your body is out of balance. Reversing hypertension naturally is possible, but it requires a clear commitment to healing the root causes. The journey ahead may not be easy, but it is absolutely worth it. Your energy, longevity, mental clarity, and freedom from medications depend on the actions you take next.

To truly get to the root of hypertension, **you must implement all seven elements presented in this book.** Each one addresses a different cause or contributor to high blood pressure. Ignoring even one may prevent full healing and leave you stuck managing symptoms rather than resolving them. These elements are not optional or interchangeable. They are interconnected, and together, they form the foundation for long-term health transformation. Below is a summary of each element with practical steps to begin applying them.

1. Food-Induced Hypertension

Begin by removing inflammatory foods from your diet. Eliminate refined carbohydrates, processed meats, added sugars, and unhealthy oils. Focus on whole, anti-inflammatory foods such as leafy greens, gluten free grains, healthy fats, and antioxidant-rich fruits. Follow the ASTR Diet principles outlined in *Eat to Heal*, and track your meals and symptoms in a journal to measure your progress.

2. Drug-Induced Hypertension

Review your current medications and supplements with a qualified healthcare provider. Some medications may be contributing to elevated blood pressure without your awareness. Identify any drugs known to increase blood pressure and discuss safer alternatives. Never discontinue medication on your own, but be proactive in working with your doctor to align your treatment plan with your health goals.

3. Vitamin, Mineral, and Hormonal Imbalances

Get tested for common nutrient and hormonal deficiencies that impact blood pressure. Work with a clinical nutritionist to create a personalized supplement and nutrition plan. Focus on correcting deficiencies in magnesium, potassium, iron, vitamin D, and B vitamins. Balanced nutrition supports cellular function, improves circulation, and restores the body's ability to regulate blood pressure naturally.

4. Medicinal Tea

Incorporate healing teas into your daily routine. Hibiscus, rooibos, chamomile, lemon balm, and green tea offer powerful cardiovascular support. Aim for one to two cups per day using organic, unsweetened options. Let this be a calming ritual that supports hydration and provides plant compounds that relax blood vessels and reduce inflammation.

5. Exercise

Start moving consistently. Choose activities you enjoy such as walking, strength training, or swimming. Begin with 20 to 30 minutes of activity most days of the week. Movement helps reduce blood pressure, strengthen your heart, improve blood flow, and lower stress hormones. Exercise is medicine, and consistency is more important than intensity.

6. Stress Management

Identify the stressors that affect your health and implement daily techniques to reduce them. Try deep breathing, prayer, journaling, gratitude, or meditation for just a few minutes each day. Chronic stress triggers a hormonal cascade that raises blood pressure. Learning to calm your nervous system is essential for long-term healing.

7. Behavioral Modification

Evaluate your habits honestly. What daily choices are working against your health? Begin replacing them with intentional behaviors that align with your goals. Improve sleep hygiene, and build structure into your routines. Use tools like habit tracking, accountability, and supportive environments to help you stay consistent.

Final Encouragement

You now have the roadmap. The information is in your hands. The question is whether you will take the next step. Reversing high blood pressure naturally is not about trying one or two strategies and hoping for results. It is about **fully committing to all seven elements** as a unified lifestyle shift. You are capable. You are not broken. Your body was designed to heal. Begin today. Choose one change, then another, and keep going. Day by day, you are building a stronger, healthier future.

Your transformation begins now.

Recommended Resources

How to Access Online Content
1. Open the camera app on your smartphone.
2. Point the camera at the barcode.
3. A notification will appear with a link. Tap the notification to open the link in your browser.

Limited Time Offer: FREE 30-minute Health Coach Consultation

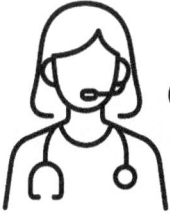

FREE
CONSULTATION
WITH
HEALTH COACH

GET STARTED

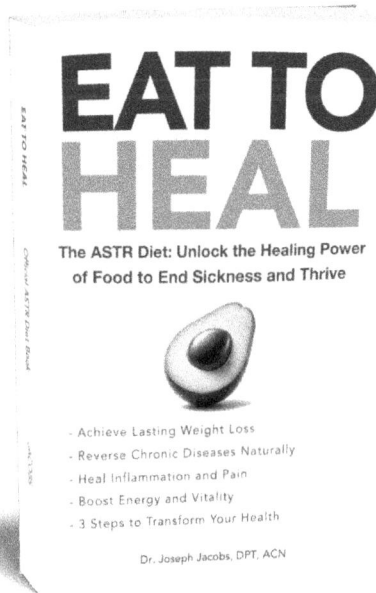

EAT TO HEAL

The ASTR Diet: Unlock the Healing Power of Food to End Sickness and Thrive

- Achieve Lasting Weight Loss
- Reverse Chronic Diseases Naturally
- Heal Inflammation and Pain
- Boost Energy and Vitality
- 3 Steps to Transform Your Health

Dr. Joseph Jacobs, DPT, ACN

BEATING ANXIETY & DEPRESSION

14 NATURAL SECRETS

BEATING
ANXIETY
&
DEPRESSION

BONUS VIDEOS

14 NATURAL SECRETS TO
A HAPPIER LIFE

- Conquer Anxiety & Depression Naturally
- Heal the Root Causes & Reclaim Your Life
- Created by a Doctor Who Conquered PTSD & Depression
- Science-Based Strategies for Lasting Change

Dr. Joseph Jacobs, DPT, ACN

BEATING MIGRAINES

7 NATURAL SECRETS

BEATING
MIGRAINES

BONUS VIDEOS

7 NATURAL SECRETS FOR
LASTING RELIEF

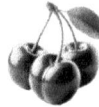

- End Migraines Naturally
- Clinically Proven Methods
- Treat the Root Cause, Not Symptoms
- Insights from a Doctor & Migraine Survivor
- Research-Backed Relief for Life

Dr. Joseph Jacobs, DPT, ACN

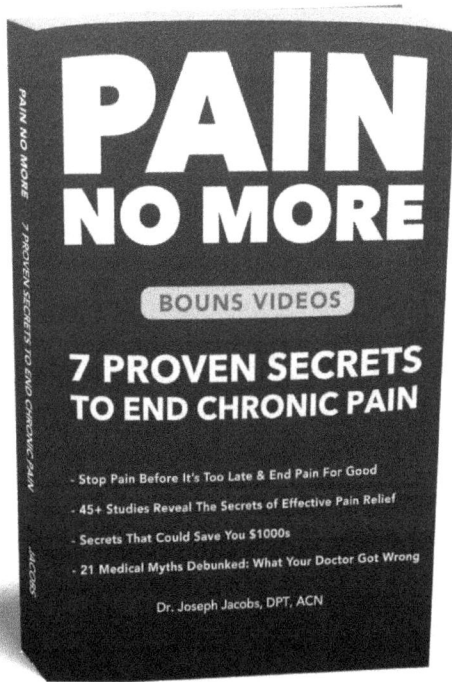

PAIN
NO MORE

BOUNS VIDEOS

7 PROVEN SECRETS
TO END CHRONIC PAIN

- Stop Pain Before It's Too Late & End Pain For Good
- 45+ Studies Reveal The Secrets of Effective Pain Relief
- Secrets That Could Save You $1000s
- 21 Medical Myths Debunked: What Your Doctor Got Wrong

Dr. Joseph Jacobs, DPT, ACN

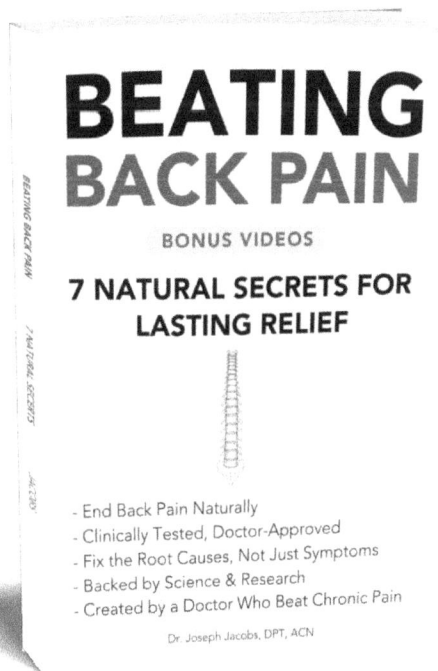

BEATING
BACK PAIN

BONUS VIDEOS

7 NATURAL SECRETS FOR
LASTING RELIEF

- End Back Pain Naturally
- Clinically Tested, Doctor-Approved
- Fix the Root Causes, Not Just Symptoms
- Backed by Science & Research
- Created by a Doctor Who Beat Chronic Pain

Dr. Joseph Jacobs, DPT, ACN

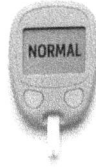

REVERSING
DIABETES
10 NATURAL SECRETS TO REVERSE
DIABETES WITHOUT DRUGS

NORMAL

- Drug-Free, Side-Effect-Free, Science-Backed Healing
- Treat the Root Cause, Not Just the Symptoms
- Proven Natural Strategies That Get Results

Dr. Joseph Jacobs, DPT, ACN

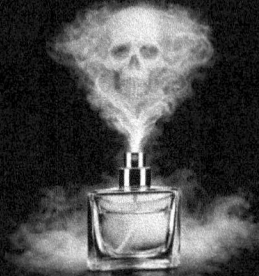

KILLED BY
FRAGRANCE
How Synthetic Scents Make Us Sick

- Exposed by peer-reviewed research
- Links everyday fragrance exposure to chronic disease
- Built on science, not opinion

Dr. Joseph Jacobs, DPT, ACN

Your

SHOES

HURT YOU

Why Does Your Pain Keep Coming
Back and *How to Fix It*

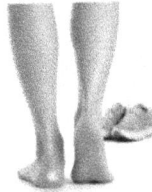

BONUS VIDEOS

- Fix Your Feet. Fix Your Pain.
- Why Modern Shoes Create Chronic Pain
- Backed by Biomechanics and Clinical Research

Dr. Joseph Jacobs, DPT, ACN

Aldosterone – A mineralocorticoid hormone produced by the adrenal cortex that regulates sodium retention and potassium excretion, influencing blood volume and pressure.

Angiotensin-Converting Enzyme (ACE) – An enzyme that converts angiotensin I to angiotensin II, a potent vasoconstrictor. ACE inhibitors are used to treat high blood pressure and heart failure.

Angiotensin II – A hormone that constricts blood vessels and stimulates aldosterone release, thereby raising blood pressure.

Antihypertensive – A class of medications used to lower elevated blood pressure, including diuretics, beta-blockers, calcium channel blockers, and ACE inhibitors.

Apoptosis – Programmed cell death, often disrupted in chronic inflammation and disease processes, including vascular dysfunction.

Arrhythmia – An abnormal heart rhythm that may be caused or worsened by electrolyte imbalances or hypertension.

Atherosclerosis – A condition in which plaque builds up in the arteries, narrowing them and increasing the risk of hypertension, stroke, and heart attack.

Autonomic Nervous System (ANS) – The part of the nervous system responsible for regulating involuntary physiological functions such as heart rate and blood pressure. Includes the sympathetic and parasympathetic branches.

Baroreceptor Reflex – A feedback mechanism in blood vessels that helps maintain blood pressure homeostasis through changes in heart rate and vessel tone.

Beta-Blocker – A type of antihypertensive drug that blocks the effects of adrenaline on the heart, slowing heart rate and reducing blood pressure.

Cardiac Output – The amount of blood the heart pumps per minute. An increase can raise blood pressure.

Cortisol – A glucocorticoid hormone released in response to stress; chronically high levels are linked to elevated blood pressure and vascular inflammation.

Cytokines – Small proteins released by immune cells that mediate and regulate immunity and inflammation. Elevated levels are associated with endothelial dysfunction and hypertension.

Diastolic Pressure – The pressure in the arteries when the heart is resting between beats. It is the bottom number in a blood pressure reading.

Diuretic – A medication that promotes the excretion of water and sodium, reducing blood volume and blood pressure.

Glossary

Endothelium – The thin layer of cells lining blood vessels that regulates vascular tone, blood flow, and inflammation. Dysfunction of the endothelium is central in hypertension.

Epigenetics – The study of how behaviors and environment can cause changes in gene expression without altering the DNA sequence; important in understanding hereditary and lifestyle-induced hypertension.

Free Radicals – Unstable molecules that damage cells through oxidative stress, contributing to vascular aging and hypertension.

Glycation – The bonding of sugar molecules to proteins or lipids, leading to oxidative damage and vascular stiffening, often seen in hypertension and diabetes.

Heart Rate Variability (HRV) – A measure of variation in time between heartbeats, reflecting autonomic nervous system balance. Low HRV is associated with stress and cardiovascular risk.

Homeostasis – The body's process of maintaining stable internal conditions, such as temperature and blood pressure.

Hypertrophy (Cardiac) – Thickening of the heart muscle, often due to prolonged hypertension, leading to reduced cardiac efficiency.

Inflammation – The body's immune response to injury or infection. Chronic inflammation contributes to arterial stiffness and hypertension.

Insulin Resistance – A condition in which cells become less responsive to insulin, often leading to elevated blood sugar and blood pressure.

Lipid Peroxidation – Oxidative degradation of lipids, a process implicated in endothelial damage and atherosclerosis.

Magnesium – A mineral critical to vascular tone and endothelial function. Deficiency can contribute to hypertension.

Mitochondria – Organelles responsible for energy production in cells; mitochondrial dysfunction is linked to hypertension and metabolic disorders.

Nitric Oxide (NO) – A vasodilator produced by endothelial cells that plays a key role in maintaining vascular tone and reducing blood pressure.

Plaque (Atheromatous) – A build-up of lipids, cholesterol, calcium, and cellular debris in the arterial wall, contributing to narrowing and stiffening of arteries.

Renin-Angiotensin-Aldosterone System (RAAS) – A hormonal system that regulates blood pressure and fluid balance. Overactivation is a major contributor to hypertension.

Sodium-Potassium Pump – A cellular mechanism that maintains fluid balance and nerve function. Imbalances can affect blood pressure regulation.

Sphygmomanometer – A device used to measure blood pressure, typically consisting of an inflatable cuff and a gauge.

Systolic Pressure – The pressure in the arteries during the contraction of the heart muscle. It is the top number in a blood pressure reading.

Vasoconstriction – Narrowing of the blood vessels, which increases blood pressure.

Vasodilation – Widening of the blood vessels, which lowers blood pressure.

Vascular Resistance – The force opposing blood flow within vessels. Higher resistance increases blood pressure.

References

1. Whelton PK, Carey RM, Aronow WS, et al. 2017 ACC/AHA/AAPA/ABC/ACPM/AGS/APhA/ ASH/ASPC/NMA/PCNA guideline for the prevention, detection, evaluation, and management of high blood pressure in adults. J Am Coll Cardiol. 2018;71(19):e127-e248.
2. Carretero OA, Oparil S. Essential hypertension. Part I: definition and etiology. Circulation. 2000;101(3):329-335.
3. Centers for Disease Control and Prevention (CDC). Facts About Hypertension. 2023. https://www.cdc.gov/bloodpressure/facts.htm
4. He FJ, MacGregor GA. A comprehensive review on salt and health and current experience of worldwide salt reduction programmes. J Hum Hypertens. 2007;21(6):717-725.
5. Johnson RJ, Segal MS, Sautin Y, et al. Potential role of sugar (fructose) in the epidemic of hypertension. Am J Clin Nutr. 2007;86(4):899-906.
6. Fuchs FD, Chambless LE, Whelton PK, et al. Alcohol consumption and the incidence of hypertension. Hypertension. 2001;37(5):1242-1250.
7. Mozaffarian D, Katan MB, Ascherio A, et al. Trans fatty acids and cardiovascular disease. N Engl J Med.2006;354(15):1601-1613.
8. Mesas AE, Leon-Munoz LM, Rodriguez-Artalejo F, Lopez-Garcia E. The effect of coffee on blood pressure. Am J Clin Nutr. 2011;94(4):1113-1126.
9. Shimomura T, Sakamoto M, Ito H, et al. MSG-induced vascular stress and hypertension risk. Nutr Neurosci.2019;22(7):490-498.
10. Aragón LE, et al. Cardiovascular impact of dairy elimination in metabolic patients. Nutr Health. 2020;26(3):217-225.
11. Sarchielli P, et al. Role of nitric oxide and arginine pathways in primary hypertension. J Hypertens. 2012;30(3):472-478.
12. Lippi G, Mattiuzzi C, Cervellin G. Hydration, electrolyte balance, and cardiovascular risk. Ann Transl Med.2020;8(23):1601.
13. El-Serag HB, Satia JA, Rabeneck L. Dietary intake and the risk of gastroesophageal reflux disease: a cross sectional study in volunteers. Am J Gastroenterol. 2005;100(5):938–945.
14. Jackson RW, Amdur RL, White LE. Inflammation and endothelial dysfunction: the link between food sensitivities and hypertension. Hypertens Res. 2018;41(10):817–825.
15. McKay DL, Chen CY, Saltzman E, Blumberg JB. Hibiscus sabdariffa L. tea (tisane) lowers blood pressure in prehypertensive and mildly hypertensive adults. J Nutr. 2010;140(2):298–303.
16. Peng X, Zhou R, Wang B, et al. Effect of green tea consumption on blood pressure: a meta-analysis of 13 randomized controlled trials. Sci Rep. 2014;4:6251.
17. Yang YC, Lu FH, Wu JS, et al. The protective effect of habitual tea consumption on hypertension. Arch Intern Med.2004;164(14):1534–1540.
18. Persson IA, Persson K, Hägg S, Andersson RG. Effects of rooibos tea on angiotensin-converting enzyme activity and blood pressure in spontaneously hypertensive rats. Public Health Nutr. 2010;13(6):730–733.
19. Amsterdam JD, Li Y, Soeller I, et al. A randomized, double-blind, placebo-controlled trial of oral Matricaria recutita (chamomile) extract therapy for generalized anxiety disorder. J Clin Psychopharmacol. 2009;29(4):378–382.
20. Kennedy DO, Scholey AB, Tildesley NT, et al. Modulation of mood and cognitive performance following acute administration of Melissa officinalis (lemon balm). Phytomedicine. 2004;11(5):375–382.
21. Kunutsor SK, Apekey TA, Steur M. Vitamin D and risk of future hypertension: meta-analysis of 283,537 participants. J Hypertens. 2013;31(12):2225–2234.

References

22. Zhang X, Li Y, Del Gobbo LC, et al. Effects of magnesium supplementation on blood pressure: a meta-analysis of randomized double-blind placebo-controlled trials. Hypertension. 2016;68(2):324–333.

23. Wilson CP, Ward M, McNulty H, et al. Riboflavin offers a targeted strategy for managing hypertension in patients with the MTHFR 677TT genotype. Hypertension. 2012;60(2):378–384.

24. Herrmann W, Obeid R, Schorr H, Geisel J. Functional vitamin B12 deficiency and determination of holotranscobalamin in populations at risk. Clin Chem Lab Med. 2007;45(12):1740–1746.

25. Verhoef P, Hennekens CH, Malinow MR, et al. A randomized trial on the effect of vitamin B6, B12 and folic acid on homocysteine and blood pressure. Am J Clin Nutr. 2002;75(1):57–63.

26. Forman JP, Rimm EB, Stampfer MJ, et al. Folate intake and the risk of incident hypertension among US women. JAMA. 2005;293(3):320–329.

27. Rosenfeldt FL, Haas SJ, Krum H, et al. Coenzyme Q10 in the treatment of hypertension: a meta-analysis of the clinical trials. J Hum Hypertens. 2007;21(4):297–306.

28. Zacharski LR, Chow BK, Howes PS, et al. Decreased cancer risk after iron reduction in patients with peripheral arterial disease. J Natl Cancer Inst. 2000;92(12):183–190.

29. Song Y, Freudenheim JL, Albanes D, et al. Zinc intake and the risk of prostate cancer: a meta-analysis of observational studies. Nutr Cancer. 2009;61(6):802–811.

30. Reckelhoff JF. Gender differences in the regulation of blood pressure. Hypertension. 2001;37(5):1199–1208.

31. Udovcic M, Pena RH, Patham B, Tabatabai L, Kansara A. Hypothyroidism and the heart. Anesth Analg.2017;125(3):904–910.

32. Whitworth JA, Williamson PM, Mangos G, Kelly JJ. Cardiovascular consequences of cortisol excess. Vasc Health Risk Manag. 2005;1(4):291–299.

33. Johnson AG, Nguyen TV, Day RO. Do nonsteroidal anti-inflammatory drugs affect blood pressure? A meta-analysis. Ann Intern Med. 2013;121(4):289–300.

34. Radack K, Deck CC. Are oral decongestants safe in hypertension? Ann Pharmacother. 1995;29(11):1126–1128.

35. Goodwin JE, Geller DS. Glucocorticoid-induced hypertension. Pediatr Nephrol. 2011;26(7):1059–1066.

36. Oparil S, Hypertension in women. J Clin Hypertens. 2005;7(3):175–182.

37. Licht CM, de Geus EJ, Seldenrijk A, et al. Depression is associated with decreased blood pressure, but antidepressant use increases the risk for hypertension. Hypertension. 2009;53(4):631–638.

38. Wilens TE, Hammerness PG, Biederman J, et al. Blood pressure changes associated with medication treatment of adults with attention-deficit/hyperactivity disorder. J Clin Psychiatry. 2005;66(2):253–259.

39. Textor SC, Canzanello VJ, Taler SJ, et al. Cyclosporine-induced hypertension after transplantation. Mayo Clin Proc. 2000;75(11):1187–1197.

40. Maitland ML, Bakris GL, Black HR, et al. Initial assessment, surveillance, and management of blood pressure in patients receiving vascular endothelial growth factor signaling pathway inhibitors. J Natl Cancer Inst.2010;102(9):596–604.

41. American Heart Association. Stress and High Blood Pressure. 2022. https://www.heart.org

42. Steptoe A, Kivimäki M. Stress and cardiovascular disease: an update on current knowledge. Hypertension.2013;62(3):331-337.

References

43. Chrousos GP. Stress and disorders of the stress system. Nat Rev Endocrinol. 2009;5(7):374-381.
44. Whitworth JA, Williamson PM, Mangos G, Kelly JJ. Cardiovascular consequences of cortisol excess. Vasc Health Risk Manag. 2005;1(4):291–299.
45. Rozanski A, Blumenthal JA, Kaplan J. Impact of psychological factors on the pathogenesis of cardiovascular disease and implications for therapy. Circulation. 2005;111(13):1717-1721.
46. Pescatello LS, MacDonald HV, Lamberti L, Johnson BT. Exercise for hypertension: a prescription update integrating existing recommendations with emerging research. Curr Hypertens Rep. 2015;17(11):87.
47. Green DJ, Maiorana A, O'Driscoll G, Taylor R. Effect of exercise training on endothelium-derived nitric oxide function in humans. J Physiol. 2004;561(Pt 1):1-25.
48. Stevens VJ, Obarzanek E, Cook NR, et al. Long-term weight loss and changes in blood pressure: results of the Trials of Hypertension Prevention, Phase II. Ann Intern Med. 2001;134(1):1-11.
49. Paluska SA, Schwenk TL. Physical activity and mental health: current concepts. Sports Med. 2000;29(3):167-180.
50. Ross R, Dagnone D, Jones PJ, et al. Reduction in obesity and related comorbid conditions after diet-induced weight loss or exercise-induced weight loss in men. Ann Intern Med. 2000;133(2):92-103.
51. Cornelissen VA, Fagard RH. Effects of endurance training on blood pressure, blood pressure–regulating mechanisms, and cardiovascular risk factors. Hypertension. 2005;46(4):667-675.
52. MacDonald HV, Johnson BT, Huedo-Medina TB, et al. Dynamic resistance training as stand-alone antihypertensive lifestyle therapy: a meta-analysis. J Am Heart Assoc. 2016;5(10):e003231.
53. Inder JD, Carlson DJ, Dieberg G, McFarlane JR, Hess NC, Smart NA. Isometric exercise training for blood pressure management: a systematic review and meta-analysis. Mayo Clin Proc. 2016;91(5):549-560.
54. Cui J, Yan JH, Yan LM, Pan L, Le JJ, Guo YZ. Effects of yoga in adults with hypertension: meta-analysis. Evid Based Complement Alternat Med. 2016;2016:1-9.
55. Appel LJ, Moore TJ, Obarzanek E, et al. A clinical trial of the effects of dietary patterns on blood pressure. N Engl J Med. 1997;336(16):1117–1124.
56. Cornelissen VA, Fagard RH. Effects of endurance training on blood pressure, blood pressure–regulating mechanisms, and cardiovascular risk factors. Hypertension. 2005;46(4):667–675.
57. Blumenthal JA, Sherwood A, Babyak MA, et al. Effects of stress management on the quality of life and blood pressure control in patients with hypertension. Arch Intern Med. 2010;170(2):113–122.
58. Palagini L, Bruno RM, Gemignani A, et al. Sleep loss and hypertension: a systematic review. Curr Pharm Des.2013;19(13):2409–2419.
59. Virdis A, Giannarelli C, Neves MF, et al. Cigarette smoking and hypertension. Curr Pharm Des.2010;16(23):2518–2525.
60. Heisler M, Vijan S, Makki F, Piette JD. Diabetes control with reciprocal peer support versus nurse care management. Ann Intern Med. 2010;153(8):507–515.
61. GBD 2016 Alcohol Collaborators. (2018). Alcohol use and burden for 195 countries and territories, 1990–2016: A systematic analysis for the Global Burden of Disease Study 2016. The Lancet, 392(10152), 1015–1035. https://doi.org/10.1016/S0140-6736(18)31310-2

References

62. Roerecke, M., Kaczorowski, J., Tobe, S. W., Gmel, G., Hasan, O. S. M., Rehm, J., & O'Donnell, M. (2017). The effect of a reduction in alcohol consumption on blood pressure: A systematic review and meta-analysis. Journal of the American Heart Association, 6(9), e006032. https://doi.org/10.1161/JAHA.117.006032

63. World Health Organization, International Agency for Research on Cancer. (2012). IARC monographs on the evaluation of carcinogenic risks to humans. Volume 100E: Personal habits and indoor combustions. https://monographs.iarc.who.int/wp-content/uploads/2018/06/mono100E.pdf

64. He FJ, Li J, MacGregor GA. Effect of longer-term modest salt reduction on blood pressure. Cochrane Database Syst Rev. 2013;(4):CD004937. doi:10.1002/14651858.CD004937.pub2

65. Rauber F, da Costa Louzada ML, Steele EM, et al. Ultra-processed food consumption and chronic non-communicable diseases-related dietary nutrient profile in the UK (2008–2014). Nutrients. 2018;10(5):587. doi:10.3390/nu10050587

66. Houston M. The role of magnesium in hypertension and cardiovascular disease. J Clin Hypertens.2011;13(11):843–847. doi:10.1111/j.1751-7176.2011.00538.x

67. Fardet A, Rock E. Ultra-processed foods and chronic diseases: a review of the current evidence. Nutrients.2021;13(8):2798. doi:10.3390/nu13082798

68. Liu S, Willett WC, Stampfer MJ, et al. A prospective study of dietary glycemic load, carbohydrate intake, and risk of coronary heart disease in US women. Am J Clin Nutr. 2000;71(6):1455–1461. doi:10.1093/ajcn/71.6.1455

69. Brown IJ, Stamler J, Van Horn L, et al. Sugar-sweetened beverage, sugar intake of individuals, and their blood pressure: International Study of Macro/Micronutrients and Blood Pressure. Hypertension. 2011;57(4):695–701. doi:10.1161/HYPERTENSIONAHA.110.157321

70. Johnson RJ, Segal MS, Sautin Y, et al. Potential role of sugar (fructose) in the epidemic of hypertension, obesity and the metabolic syndrome. Hypertension. 2007;50(2):293–301. doi:10.1161/HYPERTENSIONAHA.106.083204

71. Mozaffarian D, Katan MB, Ascherio A, Stampfer MJ, Willett WC. Trans fatty acids and cardiovascular disease. N Engl J Med. 2006;354(15):1601–1613. doi:10.1056/NEJMra054035

72. Lopez-Garcia E, Schulze MB, Manson JE, et al. Consumption of trans fatty acids is related to plasma biomarkers of inflammation and endothelial dysfunction. J Nutr. 2005;135(3):562–566. doi:10.1093/jn/135.3.562

73. Calvo MS, Uribarri J. Public health impact of dietary phosphorus excess on bone and cardiovascular health in the general population. Am J Clin Nutr. 2013;98(1):6–15. doi:10.3945/ajcn.112.053934

74. He K, Du S, Xun P, Sharma S, Wang H, Zhai F, Popkin B. Consumption of monosodium glutamate in relation to incidence of overweight in Chinese adults: China Health and Nutrition Survey (CHNS). Am J Clin Nutr.2011;93(6):1328–1336. doi:10.3945/ajcn.110.008870

75. Fardet A, Rock E. Ultra-processed foods and chronic diseases: a review of the current evidence. Nutrients.2021;13(8):2798. doi:10.3390/nu13082798

76. Wasilewska J, Kaczmarski M, Kostyra E, Kostyra H. Cow's milk allergy: a complex disorder. Nutrients. 2017;9(11):1148. doi:10.3390/nu9111148

77. Jianqin S, Leiming X, Lu X, et al. Effects of A1 and A2 beta-casein on blood pressure and inflammatory markers in humans: a randomized controlled trial. Nutrition Journal. 2016;15:35. doi:10.1186/s12937-016-0151-3

References

78. Kenney WL, Chiu P. Influence of age on thirst and fluid intake. Med Sci Sports Exerc. 2014;46(1):255–260. doi:10.1249/MSS.0b013e3182a1a68a

79. Cogswell ME, Zhang Z, Carriquiry AL, et al. Sodium and potassium intakes among US adults: NHANES 2003–2008. Am J Clin Nutr. 2012;96(3):647–657. doi:10.3945/ajcn.112.034413

80. Zhang X, Li Y, Del Gobbo LC, et al. Effects of magnesium supplementation on blood pressure: a meta-analysis of randomized double-blind placebo-controlled trials. Hypertension. 2016;68(2):324–333. doi:10.1161/HYPERTENSIONAHA.116.07664

81. Forman JP, Rimm EB, Curhan GC. Non-narcotic analgesic dose and risk of incident hypertension in US women. Hypertension. 2007;49(6):1063–1069. doi:10.1161/HYPERTENSIONAHA.107.087262

82. Johnson AG, Nguyen TV, Day RO. Do nonsteroidal anti-inflammatory drugs affect blood pressure? A meta-analysis. Ann Intern Med. 1994;121(4):289–300. doi:10.7326/0003-4819-121-4-199408150-00009

83. Gustafson F, Schor J, Muntzel M, et al. The effects of pseudoephedrine on blood pressure and heart rate in hypertensive and normotensive subjects. Am J Med. 1989;87(4):460–464. doi:10.1016/S0002-9343(89)80538-5

84. Walker BR. Glucocorticoids and cardiovascular disease. Eur J Endocrinol. 2007;157(5):545–559. doi:10.1530/EJE-07-0455

85. Souverein PC, Berard A, Van Staa TP, et al. Use of oral glucocorticoids and risk of cardiovascular and cerebrovascular disease in a population-based case-control study. Heart. 2004;90(8):859–865. doi:10.1136/hrt.2003.020180

86. Chasan-Taber L, Willett WC, Manson JE, et al. Prospective study of oral contraceptives and hypertension among women in the Nurses' Health Study. Am J Epidemiol. 1996;144(8):806–813. doi:10.1093/oxfordjournals.aje.a008990

87. Kirkman MS, Brizendine E, Somers EC, et al. Hormonal contraceptive use and the risk of cardiovascular disease in women. J Clin Hypertens. 2014;16(12):917–926. doi:10.1111/jch.12425

88. Thase ME, Entsuah AR, Rudolph RL. Venlafaxine extended release: a randomized controlled trial in patients with depression and associated anxiety. Psychosom Med. 2005;67(4):613–620. doi:10.1097/01.psy.0000170835.18680.87

89. Roose SP. Treatment of depression in patients with heart disease. CNS Drugs. 2003;17(12):927–937. doi:10.2165/00023210-200317120-00003

90. Hammerness P, Perrin J, Shelley-Abrahamson R, Wilens T. Cardiovascular risk of stimulant treatment in pediatric attention-deficit hyperactivity disorder: update and clinical recommendations. J Clin Psychiatry. 2009;70(10):1324–1335. doi:10.4088/JCP.08r04884

91. Midtvedt K, Hartmann A, Foss A, et al. Blood pressure in renal transplant recipients treated with tacrolimus or cyclosporine microemulsion in combination with mycophenolate mofetil. Am J Transplant. 2003;3(5):593–600. doi:10.1034/j.1600-6143.2003.00105.x

92. Choueiri TK, Mayer EL, Je Y, et al. Congestive heart failure risk in patients with cancer treated with bevacizumab: a meta-analysis. Lancet Oncol. 2010;11(9):817–827. doi:10.1016/S1470-2045(10)70136-3

93. McKay DL, Chen CY, Saltzman E, Blumberg JB. Hibiscus sabdariffa L. tea (tisane) lowers blood pressure in prehypertensive and mildly hypertensive adults. J Nutr. 2010;140(2):298–303. doi:10.3945/jn.109.115097

94. Serban MC, Sahebkar A, Zanchetti A, et al. Effect of sour tea (Hibiscus sabdariffa L.) on arterial hypertension: a systematic review and meta-analysis of randomized controlled trials. J Hypertens. 2015;33(6):1119–1127. doi:10.1097/HJH.0000000000000537

95. Peng X, Zhou R, Wang B, et al. Effect of green tea consumption on blood pressure: a meta-analysis of 13 randomized controlled trials. Sci Rep. 2014;4:6251. doi:10.1038/srep06251

96. Khalesi S, Sun J, Buys N, Jayasinghe R. Green tea catechins and blood pressure: a systematic review and meta-analysis of randomized controlled trials. Eur J Nutr. 2014;53(6):1299–1311. doi:10.1007/s00394-014-0663-9

97. Yang YC, Lu FH, Wu JS, Wu CH, Chang CJ. The protective effect of habitual tea consumption on hypertension. Arch Intern Med. 2004;164(14):1534–1540. doi:10.1001/archinte.164.14.1534

98. Zhang Y, Zhang DZ. Habitual oolong tea drinking and risk of hypertension in the Chinese population. Clin Exp Hypertens. 2011;33(5):320–326. doi:10.3109/10641963.2010.547835

99. Persson IA, Persson K, Hagg S, Andersson RG. Effects of rooibos tea (Aspalathus linearis) on angiotensin-converting enzyme activity and blood pressure in vivo and in vitro. J Ethnopharmacol. 2010;131(1):121–127. doi:10.1016/j.jep.2010.06.033

100. Amsterdam JD, Li Y, Soeller I, Rockwell K, Mao JJ, Shults J. A randomized, double-blind, placebo-controlled trial of oral Matricaria recutita (chamomile) extract therapy for generalized anxiety disorder. J Clin Psychopharmacol.2009;29(4):378–382. doi:10.1097/JCP.0b013e3181ac935c

101. Kennedy DO, Scholey AB, Tildesley NT, Perry EK, Wesnes KA. Modulation of mood and cognitive performance following acute administration of Melissa officinalis (lemon balm). Phytomedicine. 2004;11(7-8):632–638. doi:10.1016/j.phymed.2003.07.013

102. Kunutsor SK, Apekey TA, Steur M. Vitamin D and risk of future hypertension: meta-analysis of 283,537 participants. Eur J Epidemiol. 2013;28(3):205–221. doi:10.1007/s10654-013-9790-2

103. Beveridge LA, Struthers AD, Khan F, et al. Effect of vitamin D supplementation on blood pressure: a systematic review and meta-analysis incorporating individual patient data. JAMA Intern Med. 2015;175(5):745–754. doi:10.1001/jamainternmed.2015.0237

104. Zhang X, Li Y, Del Gobbo LC, et al. Effects of magnesium supplementation on blood pressure: a meta-analysis of randomized double-blind placebo-controlled trials. Hypertension. 2016;68(2):324–333. doi:10.1161/HYPERTENSIONAHA.116.07664

105. Rosanoff A, Weaver CM, Rude RK. Suboptimal magnesium status in the United States: are the health consequences underestimated? Nutr Rev. 2012;70(3):153–164. doi:10.1111/j.1753-4887.2011.00465.x

106. Wilson CP, Ward M, McNulty H, et al. Riboflavin offers a targeted strategy for managing hypertension in patients with the MTHFR 677TT genotype: a 4-year follow-up. Hypertension. 2012;60(2):379–387. doi:10.1161/HYPERTENSIONAHA.112.194340

107. Herrmann W, Obeid R, Schorr H, Geisel J. Functional vitamin B12 deficiency and determination of holotranscobalamin in populations at risk. Clin Chem Lab Med. 2003;41(11):1478–1488. doi:10.1515/CCLM.2003.227

108. den Elzen WPJ, Westendorp RGJ, Frolich M, de Ruijter W, Assendelft WJJ, Gussekloo J. Vitamin B12 and folate and the risk of anemia in old age: the Leiden 85-plus study. Arch Intern Med. 2008;168(20):2238–2244. doi:10.1001/archinte.168.20.2238

109. Verhoef P, Stampfer MJ, Buring JE, Gaziano JM, Allen RH, Stabler SP. Homocysteine metabolism and risk of hypertension: a prospective study in men. Circulation. 2002;105(13):1396–1401. doi:10.1161/01.CIR.0000012530.24310.45

110. Forman JP, Rimm EB, Stampfer MJ, Curhan GC. Folate intake and the risk of incident hypertension among US women. JAMA. 2005;293(3):320–329. doi:10.1001/jama.293.3.320

References

111. Rosenfeldt FL, Haas SJ, Krum H, et al. Coenzyme Q10 in the treatment of hypertension: a meta-analysis of the clinical trials. J Hum Hypertens. 2007;21(4):297–306. doi:10.1038/sj.jhh.1002138

112. Ho MJ, Yeung L, Samuel M. Coenzyme Q10 for hypertension. Cochrane Database Syst Rev.2016;2016(11):CD007435. doi:10.1002/14651858.CD007435.pub2

113. Zacharski LR, Chow BK, Howes PS, et al. Reduction of iron stores and cardiovascular outcomes in patients with peripheral arterial disease: a randomized controlled trial. JAMA. 2000;293(4):475–482. doi:10.1001/jama.283.4.475

114. Song Y, Wang L, Pittas AG, et al. Blood levels of zinc and magnesium are associated with cardiovascular mortality in U.S. adults. Nutr Metab Cardiovasc Dis. 2009;19(10):767–773. doi:10.1016/j.numecd.2008.10.007

115. Reckelhoff JF. Gender differences in the regulation of blood pressure. Hypertension. 2001;37(5):1199–1208. doi:10.1161/01.HYP.37.5.1199

116. Udovcic M, Pena RH, Patham B, Tabatabai L, Kansara A. Hypothyroidism and the heart. Methodist Debakey Cardiovasc J. 2017;13(2):55–59. doi:10.14797/mdcj-13-2-55

117. Whitworth JA, Williamson PM, Mangos G, Kelly JJ. Cardiovascular consequences of cortisol excess. Vasc Health Risk Manag. 2005;1(4):291–299.

118. Ghiadoni, L., Taddei, S., & Virdis, A. (2008). Endothelial function and hypertension. Current Opinion in Nephrology and Hypertension, 17(2), 105–111. https://doi.org/10.1097/MNH.0b013e3282f5285c

119. Libby, P., Ridker, P. M., & Hansson, G. K. (2011). Progress and challenges in translating the biology of atherosclerosis. Nature, 473(7347), 317–325. https://doi.org/10.1038/nature10146

120. Williams, B., Mancia, G., Spiering, W., Agabiti Rosei, E., Azizi, M., Burnier, M., ... & Tsioufis, K. (2018). 2018 ESC/ESH Guidelines for the management of arterial hypertension. European Heart Journal, 39(33), 3021–3104. https://doi.org/10.1093/eurheartj/ehy339

121. Green DJ, Hopman MT, Padilla J, Laughlin MH, Thijssen DH. Vascular adaptation to exercise in humans: role of hemodynamic stimuli. Physiol Rev. 2017;97(2):495-528. doi:10.1152/physrev.00014.2016

122. Supports the role of the endothelium in regulating vascular tone and the effects of nitric oxide.

123. Ghiadoni L, Taddei S, Virdis A. Endothelial function and hypertension. Curr Opin Nephrol Hypertens. 2012;21(3):256-261. doi:10.1097/MNH.0b013e3283511f6b

124. Describes how endothelial dysfunction is an early marker in the development of hypertension.

125. Deanfield JE, Halcox JP, Rabelink TJ. Endothelial function and dysfunction: testing and clinical relevance. Circulation.2007;115(10):1285-1295. doi:10.1161/CIRCULATIONAHA.106.652859

126. Reviews the clinical relevance of endothelial dysfunction in cardiovascular disease.

127. Schmidt A, Hammann F, Längin M, et al. The impact of dietary polyphenols on vascular health—A review. Nutrients.2020;12(3):856. doi:10.3390/nu12030856

128. Supports the protective effects of nutrition (e.g., polyphenols) on endothelial health.

129. Higashi Y, Noma K, Yoshizumi M, Kihara Y. Endothelial function and oxidative stress in cardiovascular diseases. Circ J.2009;73(3):411-418. doi:10.1253/circj.CJ-08-1102

130. Green DJ, Hopman MT, Padilla J, Laughlin MH, Thijssen DH. Vascular adaptation to exercise in humans: role of hemodynamic stimuli. Physiol Rev. 2017;97(2):495-528. doi:10.1152/physrev.00014.2016

References

131. Ghiadoni L, Taddei S, Virdis A. Endothelial function and hypertension. Curr Opin Nephrol Hypertens.2012;21(3):256-261. doi:10.1097/MNH.0b013e3283511f6b

132. Deanfield JE, Halcox JP, Rabelink TJ. Endothelial function and dysfunction: testing and clinical relevance. Circulation. 2007;115(10):1285-1295. doi:10.1161/CIRCULATIONAHA.106.652859

133. Higashi Y, Noma K, Yoshizumi M, Kihara Y. Endothelial function and oxidative stress in cardiovascular diseases. Circ J. 2009;73(3):411-418. doi:10.1253/circj.CJ-08-1102

134. Zhang Y, Vittinghoff E, Pletcher MJ, et al. Associations of inflammatory markers with endothelial function in young adults. Circulation. 2014;130(14):1110-1116. doi:10.1161/CIRCULATIONAHA.113.007288

135. Schmidt A, Hammann F, Längin M, et al. The impact of dietary polyphenols on vascular health—A review. Nutrients. 2020;12(3):856. doi:10.3390/nu12030856

136. Higashi Y, Noma K, Yoshizumi M, Kihara Y. Endothelial function and oxidative stress in cardiovascular diseases. Circ J.2009;73(3):411-418. doi:10.1253/circj.CJ-08-1102

137. Ghiadoni L, Taddei S, Virdis A. Endothelial function and hypertension. Curr Opin Nephrol Hypertens. 2012;21(3):256-261. doi:10.1097/MNH.0b013e3283511f6b

138. Bautista LE, Vera LM, Arenas IA, Gamarra G. Independent association between inflammatory markers (C-reactive protein, interleukin-6, and TNF-alpha) and essential hypertension. J Hum Hypertens. 2005;19(2):149-154. doi:10.1038/sj.jhh.1001785

139. Harrison DG, Guzik TJ, Lob HE, et al. Inflammation, immunity, and hypertension. Hypertension. 2011;57(2):132-140. doi:10.1161/HYPERTENSIONAHA.110.163576

140. Sesso HD, Buring JE, Rifai N, Blake GJ, Gaziano JM, Ridker PM. C-reactive protein and the risk of developing hypertension. JAMA. 2003;290(22):2945-2951. doi:10.1001/jama.290.22.2945

141. Esposito K, Giugliano D. The impact of diet and lifestyle on vascular inflammation in hypertension. J Hum Hypertens.2004;18(8):487-494. doi:10.1038/sj.jhh.1001712

142. Elliott P, Stamler J, Nichols R, et al. Intersalt revisited: further analyses of 24 hour sodium excretion and blood pressure within and across populations. BMJ. 1996;312(7041):1249-1253. doi:10.1136/bmj.312.7041.1249

143. Aburto NJ, Hanson S, Gutierrez H, Hooper L, Elliott P, Cappuccio FP. Effect of increased potassium intake on cardiovascular risk factors and disease: systematic review and meta-analyses. BMJ. 2013;346:f1378. doi:10.1136/bmj.f1378

144. Engel GL. The need for a new medical model: a challenge for biomedicine. *Science*. 1977;196(4286):129-136.

145. Appel LJ, Champagne CM, Harsha DW, et al. Effects of comprehensive lifestyle modification on blood pressure control: main results of the PREMIER clinical trial. *JAMA*. 2003;289(16):2083-2093.
146. Lane MM, Davis JA, Beattie S, et al. Ultra-processed food consumption and cardiometabolic health outcomes: umbrella review. *BMJ*. 2024;384:e077310.
147. Jayalath VH, de Souza RJ, Ha V, et al. Sugar-sweetened beverage consumption and incident hypertension: a systematic review and meta-analysis of prospective cohorts. *Am J Clin Nutr*. 2015;102(4):914-921.
148. Aburto NJ, Hanson S, Gutierrez H, Hooper L, Elliott P, Cappuccio FP. Effect of increased potassium intake on cardiovascular risk factors and disease: systematic review and meta-analyses. *BMJ*. 2013;346:f1378.
149. Soltani S, Shirani F, Chitsazi MJ, et al. Mediterranean diet and blood pressure: systematic review and meta-analysis of randomized controlled trials. *Nutr Metab Cardiovasc Dis*. 2024.
150. Pope JE, Anderson JJ, Felson DT. A meta-analysis of the effects of nonsteroidal anti-inflammatory drugs on blood pressure. *Arch Intern Med*. 1993;153(4):477-484.
151. Ruschitzka F, Borer JS, Krum H, et al. Differential blood pressure effects of ibuprofen, naproxen, and celecoxib in patients with arthritis (PRECISION-ABPM). *Eur Heart J*. 2017;38(44):3282-3292.
152. Liu H, Yao J, Wang W, Zhang D. Association between duration of oral contraceptive use and risk of hypertension: a meta-analysis. *J Clin Hypertens (Greenwich)*. 2017;19(10):1032-1041.
153. Ellis AA, Sedehizadeh S, Mirmiran P, et al. Hibiscus sabdariffa and blood pressure: systematic review and meta-analysis. *Nutr Metab Cardiovasc Dis*. 2022.
154. Xu R, Yang K, Ding J, et al. Effect of green tea supplementation on blood pressure: meta-analysis of randomized trials. *Medicine (Baltimore)*. 2020.
155. Mahdavi-Roshan M, Salari A, Ghorbani Z, Ashouri A. Effects of regular consumption of green or black tea on blood pressure in those with elevated BP or hypertension: systematic review and meta-analysis. *Clin Nutr*. 2020.
156. Benjamim CJR, Porto AA, Valenti VE, et al. Nitrate derived from beetroot juice lowers blood pressure in patients with arterial hypertension: systematic review and meta-analysis. *Front Nutr*. 2022;9:823039.
157. Zhang X, Li Y, Del Gobbo LC, Rosanoff A, Wang J, Zhang W. Effects of magnesium supplementation on blood pressure: meta-analysis of randomized trials. *Hypertension*. 2016.
158. Meng R, et al. Impact of vitamin D supplementation on blood pressure: umbrella review. *Clin Ther*. 2023.
159. Bouillon R, Marcocci C, Carmeliet G, et al. The health effects of vitamin D supplementation: evidence from human studies. *Nat Rev Endocrinol*. 2022.
160. Lin LY, et al. Universal screening for primary aldosteronism in hypertension. *Hypertension*. 2025.
161. Huang M, et al. Global prevalence and cardiovascular risk of primary aldosteronism: systematic review and meta-analysis. *Clin Endocrinol*. 2024.
162. Ye Y, Xie H, Zeng Y, et al. Association between subclinical hypothyroidism and blood pressure: meta-analysis. *Endocr Pract*. 2014.
163. Kim J, et al. Association between subclinical hypothyroidism and hypertension risk: systematic review and meta-analysis. *J Clin Med*. 2021.
164. Cornelissen VA, Smart NA. Exercise training for blood pressure: systematic review and meta-analysis. *J Am Heart Assoc*. 2013;2:e004473.
165. Lee EKP, et al. Mindfulness-based stress reduction and blood pressure: meta-analysis of randomized controlled trials. *Hypertension*. 2020.
166. Mir IA, et al. Effect of mindfulness-based meditation on blood pressure: systematic review and meta-analysis. *Complement Ther Med*. 2024.

167. Wang Q, Xi B, Liu M, Zhang Y, Fu M. Short sleep duration is associated with hypertension risk among adults: systematic review and meta-analysis. *Hypertens Res.* 2012.
168. Cappuccio FP, Kerry SM, Forbes L, Donald A. Blood pressure control by home monitoring: meta-analysis of randomized trials. *BMJ.* 2004;329(7458):145.
169. Borrell-Carrió F, Suchman AL, Epstein RM. The biopsychosocial model 25 years later: principles, practice, and scientific inquiry. *Ann Fam Med.* 2004;2(6):576–582. doi:10.1370/afm.245
170. Whelton PK, Carey RM, Aronow WS, et al. 2017 ACC/AHA guideline for the prevention, detection, evaluation, and management of high blood pressure in adults. *Hypertension.* 2018;71(6):e13–e115. doi:10.1161/HYP.0000000000000065
171. Mancia G, Grassi G. The autonomic nervous system and hypertension. *Circ Res.* 2014;114(11):1804–1814. doi:10.1161/CIRCRESAHA.114.302524
172. Spruill TM. Chronic psychosocial stress and hypertension. *Curr Hypertens Rep.* 2010;12(1):10–16. doi:10.1007/s11906-009-0084-8
173. Carney RM, Freedland KE. Depression and coronary heart disease. *Nat Rev Cardiol.* 2017;14(3):145–155. doi:10.1038/nrcardio.2016.181
174. Kaplan NM. Primary hypertension: pathogenesis. In: Kaplan's Clinical Hypertension. 11th ed. Wolters Kluwer; 2015.
175. Brook RD, Appel LJ, Rubenfire M, et al. Beyond medications and diet: alternative approaches to lowering blood pressure. *Hypertension.* 2013;61(6):1360–1383. doi:10.1161/HYP.0b013e318293645f

www.ingramcontent.com/pod-product-compliance
Lightning Source LLC
Chambersburg PA
CBHW052024030426

42335CB00026B/3270